Protect Yourself from Legionnaires' Disease

The waterborne illness that continues to kill and harm

Matthew R. Freije

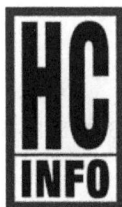

HC INFO

Protect Yourself from Legionnaires' Disease
The waterborne illness that continues to kill and harm

by Matthew R. Freije

Cover photo of woman washing her face. © Andres Rodriguez, Dreamstime.com
Cover photo of enjoying a hot tub. © Glenda Powers, Dreamstime.com
Cover photo of fountain in Bucharest. © Radu Coriu, Dreamstime.com
Cover photo of *Legionella pneumophila*, © Sebastian Kaulitzki. Dreamstime.com

Copy editing by Robin Quinn

Published by:
HC Information Resources Inc.
Solona Beach, CA, USA
+1-760-494-3063
hcinfo@hcinfo.com
http://hcinfo.com

ISBN 1-930488-17-3 or 978-1-930488-17-5 (softcover)

Acknowledgments

The scientific evidence on which this book is based was generated by numerous individuals who have devoted years of their lives to *Legionella* research. Some of the book is composed of information excerpted from my first book, *Legionellae Control in Health Care Facilities: A Guide for Minimizing Risk*, and two reports, the manuscripts of which were reviewed for technical accuracy by several colleagues who graciously contributed their time and knowledge.

Warning and disclaimer

Contents

1. What you need to know about Legionnaires' disease

Reports of a strange illness began pouring in to the Pennsylvania (USA) Department of Health in late July 1976. By August 2, the department realized that all of the reports involved persons who had attended the 58th annual convention of the American Legion's Pennsylvania Chapter held at the Bellevue-Stratford Hotel in Philadelphia from July 21st to 24th. Illness struck 221 persons, 72 of whom did not attend the convention but were in or near the Bellevue-Stratford Hotel over the same period. Of the 221, 34 died.

Then began one of the largest epidemic investigations in history. After months of searching, investigators traced the illness, which had been named "Legionnaires' disease" by the press, to a previously unknown bacterium now called *Legionella*.

Legionella had actually been causing disease for decades. The first known hospital outbreak occurred in 1965 when 81 patients at St. Elizabeth's Hospital in

Washington, DC (USA) developed pneumonia and 14 died. The cause could not be found. Twelve years later, however, after *Legionella* was discovered, frozen specimens retained from the outbreak were removed from storage and retested. The results confirmed that *Legionella* was the cause.

Much has been learned about how to prevent Legionnaires' disease since the Philadelphia outbreak and the subsequent discovery of *Legionella.* Sadly, though, the disease kills about as many people today as in the past, due in part to lack of preventive action.

Legionella

Legionella is a type of bacteria found primarily in water, although researchers have also found it in potting soils. About 50 species of *Legionella* have been identified by laboratory workers. Some species have more than one serogroup, and some serogroups have several subtypes. For example, the *Legionella* species *pneumophila* has 15 serogroups, and *Legionella pneumophila* serogroup 1 has at least 50 subtypes.

Think of it like fruit:

> There are many varieties of fruit—grapes, apples, peaches, oranges, mangos—and there are many types of bacteria, including *Legionella*, *Pseudomonas*, *Campylobacter*, *Acinetobacter*, and *Burkholderia*.

> There are many varieties of grapes, one of which is *Vitis vinifera*, and there are about 50 species

of *Legionella* including *pneumophila, micdadei, bozemanni, dumoffii,* and *longbeachae.*

There are two types of *Vitis vinifera* grapes, red and white, and there are 15 serogroups of *Legionella pneumophila*, identified as serogroups 1-15.

There are many types of *Vitis vinifera* red and white grapes, and there are about 50 subtypes of *Legionella pneumophila* serogroup 1.

Fewer than half of the species of *Legionella* have been linked to disease. Studies indicate that in the United States and Europe, well over 90% of community-acquired Legionnaires' cases are caused by a single species, *Legionella pneumophila*, and most (88%) by just one of its 15 serogroups, *Legionella pneumophila* serogroup 1. In Australia, however, *Legionella longbeachae* has been responsible for 51% of reported cases and *Legionella pneumophila* for only about 6%. Other *Legionella* species that have caused numerous cases of disease are *micdadei, bozemanni, dumoffii,* and *feeleii.*

Legionellosis is any illness caused by exposure to *Legionella* bacteria. The two types of legionellosis are Pontiac fever, a flu-like illness that lasts up to five days but does not require hospitalization, and Legionnaires' disease, a deadly type of pneumonia.

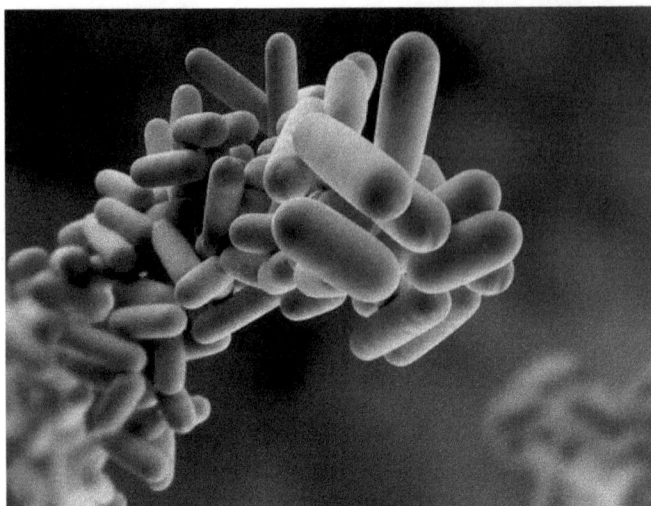

Legionella pneumophila
© Sebastian Kaulitzki. Dreamstime.com.

Symptoms of Legionnaires' disease

Symptoms of Legionnaires' disease—which appear usually within two to ten days after exposure to Legionella bacteria—may include loss of energy, headache, nausea, aching muscles, fever exceeding 40°C (104°F), chest pains, and confusion.

The severity ranges from a mild cough to a rapidly fatal pneumonia. Death occurs through progressive pneumonia with respiratory failure, shock, and multi-organ failure.

An early diagnosis and prompt treatment with an appropriate antibiotic will increase the chances of survival. Unfortunately, many who do survive

Legionnaires' experience prolonged physical and psychological impairment.

Tests required for diagnosis

Specialized laboratory tests are required to identify Legionnaires' disease. Three types of tests are used: blood tests, urine tests, and sputum tests.

Sputum tests are the most sensitive and reliable, because *Legionella*, if in the sputum, can actually be grown (cultured) in the laboratory. Seven to ten days are required for results.

Urine tests are not as accurate as sputum cultures and detect only one *Legionella* serogroup. However, lab results can be produced within 24 hours, and with some technologies, in only 15 minutes.

Blood tests require two samples with a considerable time delay between them: the first sample is drawn at the time of exposure or onset of symptoms, and the second is taken six to eight weeks later. By the time the physician receives the results, the patient has either recovered or died. Blood tests are also the least sensitive of the three methods.

A positive sputum culture confirms the disease beyond a reasonable doubt. Blood and urine tests can be "strongly positive" or "positive but not conclusive." None of the tests is totally sensitive, so the disease cannot be ruled out even if one or more of the tests is negative.

The problem of undetected cases

Legionnaires' disease is not rare. It is perceived as rare only because most cases go undetected, and because not all detected cases are reported to public health authorities. Even when cases are detected, the public rarely hears about them. Most cases—at least 65% to 80% in the United States and the United Kingdom—occur sporadically, one or two at a time. Only a small percentage of cases occur as part of the multi-case outbreaks reported by the media. The disease is seldom publicized even when lawsuits are involved because most Legionnaires' lawsuits are settled under terms of confidentiality.

All these factors make estimating disease incidence difficult. According to the Centers for Disease Control and Prevention (CDC) in Atlanta, GA (USA), between 8,000 and 18,000 people are hospitalized with Legionnaires' disease each year in the United States. However, because of cases undiagnosed or unreported, the actual number of cases could be much higher. Some have estimated as high as 100,000 annual US cases.

A case of Legionnaires' disease will go undiagnosed unless one of the special laboratory tests discussed above is performed to identify *Legionella* bacteria. Unfortunately, these tests are not routinely used, either because a test is not ordered by a physician, or is unavailable.

The CDC has estimated that only 10% of Legionnaires' cases are diagnosed, even among patients who contract it while in the hospital. Of the cases contracted anywhere other than in a hospital—such as during a hotel stay or while using a whirlpool spa—fewer than 5% are detected.

Unrecognized Legionnaires' cases are classified merely as "pneumonia with no apparent cause" (atypical pneumonia). No one knows exactly how many cases of Legionnaires' disease go unrecognized each year, but the number could be significant considering that no cause is found for almost half of the adult pneumonia cases that occur each year in the United States.

Why is undetected Legionnaires' disease such a big problem? First, untreated cases are more likely to result in death (see "*Death rate*" section at the end of this chapter). Second, if *Legionella* is not recognized as the cause of illness, no investigation is conducted to pinpoint and disinfect the source (for instance, a plumbing system), so the same contaminated water system remains a threat to other lives. Moreover, the decedent's survivors never know that the cause of death was *Legionella* and that proper water system management could have prevented it.

How Legionnaires' disease is contracted

Legionnaires' disease is contracted by inhaling small water droplets contaminated with *Legionella* bacteria or by accidentally choking the bacteria into the lungs while drinking. People can be infected with *Legionella* while washing their hands or face, brushing their teeth, showering, walking by a decorative fountain, bathing in a whirlpool spa, drinking from a water fountain, or inhaling mist emitted from a cooling tower (a water cooling device typically located on the roofs of large buildings or on platforms next to them).

Inhaling water droplets sprayed from windshield washers may be another way of contracting Legionnaires' disease, according to a study published in the June 2010 issue of the *European Journal of Epidemiology*.

The disease is entirely environmental—water is the source. It is not contagious.

According to the World Health Organization, outbreak data indicates that a low number of *Legionella* organisms are required for infection. Infection depends on the *Legionella* concentration in the water, the efficiency of the transmission of *Legionella* from the water to air, the "strength" of the particular *Legionella* strain, and the susceptibility of the person exposed.

Individuals who are most susceptible

Young and healthy nonsmokers can get Legionnaires' disease but persons who are immunocompromised or elderlyare at a much higher risk.

Organ transplant recipients are in the highest risk category. Others at high risk are people with underlying illness (diabetes), patients who have had recent surgery, and patients receiving chemotherapy, immune-suppressing steroids, mechanical ventilation, or respiratory therapy.

Smokers are at a much higher risk for contracting Legionnaires' disease. This is in part because their smoke-damaged respiratory tracts fail to keep foreign substances (water particles) out of the lungs.

In general, persons over 65 years of age and individuals with a history of heavy drinking or respiratory ailments are also at a higher risk. Men are more likely than women to get the disease.

Children have contracted Legionnaires' disease. Most of the cases have occurred in newborns following surgery, in immunosuppressed children, or through the use of *Legionella*-contaminated ventilators. In December 2007, however, 11 infants discharged in good condition from a private hospital in Cyprus had to be admitted a few days later to an intensive care unit because of Legionnaires' disease that was apparently contracted at the hospital. Three of the babies died. Reports indicated that portable ultrasonic humidifiers were the source of contamination.

Death rate

Underlying disease and advanced age not only increase the risk of contracting Legionnaires' disease but also the risk of dying from it.

People who are diagnosed soon after infection and treated with the right antibiotics are much more likely to survive. According to the World Health Organization, the death rate may be as high as 40-80% for immune-suppressed people who do not receive treatment and 5-30% for those who do.

As mentioned above ("*The problem of undetected cases*"), only a small percentage of Legionnaires' cases are detected. In some instances, even when the disease is diagnosed, it is too late. For example, according to August 2009 news reports, a 46-year-old UK woman who contracted Legionnaires' disease was initially misdiagnosed with swine flu (H1N1) and thus told by an ambulance crew that she did not need hospitalization. The ambulance crew was called two days later but again refused to take her to the hospital. She ended up getting to the hospital that day, but died four days later.

2. Survivor stories

Other than some minor spelling and grammar corrections, these are the words of the survivors, verbatim from emails and letters received over the last few years.

On 26 September 1999, my wife was placed on a respirator where she remained for nearly four weeks. She almost succumbed to the effects of multi-organ dysfunction caused by toxic Legionella pneumonia. Fortunately, from the outset, her chances for survival were greatly increased because of the infection control and pulmonary physicians correctly diagnosed her condition and immediately treated her for Legionnaires' disease. Their diagnosis was confirmed by subsequent laboratory analyses. My wife is at home now continuing to recover from this illness, which made her an in-patient for two months. The experience was harrowing for us all. ~ **J. E.**

I have recently contracted Legionnaires'.

I am an independent contractor/project manager building cellular wireless sites throughout the world. In April 2001, I accepted a contract with [company] to manage a test overlay in Phoenix, AZ. A warehouse was procured for staging of the cell-site radio equipment. I firmly believe this warehouse was the source of the bacteria as it utilized a swamp cooling system and the warehouse was empty and without power for quite some time.

On April 26, 2001, I began working in this warehouse, with no electricity turned on yet. On Monday April 30th, in the early afternoon, I was hanging "white" boards on the wall in the front office of this warehouse when the power to the building was turned on. I was on a ladder directly in front of the cooling duct when the swamp cooler came on with the electricity. I was inundated with the initial blast of stagnant smelling air. I continued working that day feeling okay.

On Tuesday May 1st, I continued a full day at the warehouse. That evening, I developed a cough, which progressed day by day. On Wednesday the 2nd, flu symptoms began along with the cough. On Thursday, I went to [the hospital] emergency. They advised me that it looked like pneumonia and advised me to check in to the hospital. I declined and asked for an antibiotics prescription and left.

I went without sleep all Thursday night, unable to breathe properly. On Friday [May 4th] at 6 a.m., I went back to the emergency room almost unable to breathe. That is pretty much all I remember until I awoke on June 3rd. My wife advised me that I was on life support for almost a month and it looked very grim at times.

Unable to walk, groom, bathe, or take care of myself in any way, I was transferred to the "REHAB" unit on June 4th where I spent the next three and a half weeks. Under extensive occupational, physical and speech therapy, I made substantial progress and was released on June 22nd with outpatient continuum three times a week for speech and physical therapy.

Matt, as a result of this Godforsaken disease, I have lost my job and will not be able to return to work until possibly August sometime. As an independent contractor, I carried no short or long term disability insurance. I have contacted the state of Arizona disease center to test this warehouse as an attempt to avert anyone else from contracting this disease and to recoup lost wages from the parties responsible for upkeep on this property. The state of Arizona advised me that they will not dispatch anyone to inspect the warehouse as I am still alive. If I would have died, the state might have sent someone to investigate. What kind of an oxymoron is that?

I have exhausted all avenues of response except for the media. Again, Matt, this disease almost killed me and I will NEVER let this go. It is my personal crusade to have the local/federal government investigate EVERY occurrence of this disease.

Any advice, suggestions, or help you can offer is greatly appreciated. ~ **T. C., July 5, 2001**

I had LD in 1997: Unconscious, fever 107 degrees F, several days on a cooling blanket, 56 days in coma, 71 days in hospital, had to learn to walk again. My neurological system is severely damaged. I am unable to work. I am fighting Social Security for disability benefits. I need some good reputable documentation of LD and its impact on the neurological system. HELP! ~ **Rowland Hatfield**

Four years ago in Miami, in a hotel whirlpool spa, I think, I caught Legionnaires' disease. It mimicked the symptoms of food poisoning, so I was treated for that. By the time I arrived home, I was very ill and admitted to the hospital. Three weeks later, they got the results of the blood tests and found *Legionella*. Treated with the right antibiotics, I got better. But I still suffer a lot, and [had I not been] … a nonsmoker and very fit (a swimmer), it would have killed me, although sometimes I wish it had … as each year I get worse. ~ **S. Finnegan, July 2002**

Many thanks to Mechele Cooper for permission to use the following excerpts from her Kennebec Journal article about Erin Doyle's amazing recovery from Legionnaires' disease.

CHELSEA [Maine] – Cathy Doyle wasn't about to let doctors pull the plug on her daughter.

Erin Doyle had contracted Legionnaires' pneumonia in September 2006 while at the Maine Medical Center in Portland.

Erin Doyle, 27, had been on dialysis and had received a kidney from her best friend, Audrey Hustus, of Gardiner. The kidney lasted for about a year and a half until Doyle's body rejected the donated organ.
Doctors were trying to save the kidney when she contracted Legionnaires' pneumonia.

"I had been there for a month, but it wasn't until October that I showed signs of (Legionnaires' pneumonia) and then I got sick really quickly," Erin Doyle said. "They put me on a ventilator. I know that it was Oct. 25 because it was my birthday. That's the day they told my parents that it wasn't good.

"By Thanksgiving, the doctor came into my room and told my parents that there was absolutely no hope of me waking up. They wanted to disconnect me, but I guess my mom came unglued at the doctor and said, 'You don't know my daughter. She's going to walk out of here.'"

Doyle did walk, or rather was wheeled out, of the hospital after being in a coma for 21 weeks.

Her physical therapist, Wendy Claveau, said Doyle is a special patient. And because of all that she has accomplished, she will receive the Overcoming Barriers Award on Sept. 26 during a luncheon at Granite Hill Estates.

Doyle said doctors kept trying to get her mother to turn off the ventilator.

"They wanted me to unplug her and I fought with the doctors," Cathy Doyle said. "They thought I wasn't facing reality, but it was my daughter and I just felt I would know that there was no hope and she was gone. I knew that she would pull through."

Doyle fought for her daughter right up until January, when she started to show signs of improving.

She kept on getting better so doctors woke her up from the drug-induced coma. Doyle was on a ventilator that took over the work of her breathing. A tube was placed from her mouth into her airways. She said doctors sedated her so she wouldn't struggle and pull the tube out, which is irritating and uncomfortable.

They told her she would have to live with the tracheotomy to help her breathe, but that came out six weeks later. They also told Doyle her voice would never be the same, but it is.

They sent her home with an oxygen tank and said she would have to use it to breathe 24 hours a day for the rest of her life.

"They were wrong there too," she said. "I'm only on it at night. All the doctors at Maine Medical Center treated me at one point or another. It was my understanding that I was the sickest patient in the hospital. It's very rare to get Legionnaires' pneumonia so none of my doctors ever treated it before. They used it as a learning tool."

Doyle came home in May 2007. After being in a coma for so long, she had to relearn how to read, write, and walk.

Therapists came to her home for the first 11 months. She now goes once a week to the Center for Health & Rehabilitation in Augusta, part of Maine General Medical Center.

Claveau said the award Doyle will receive was developed by the Maine General's rehabilitation department ...

"Erin's gone from a coma to wheelchair-based and now she's walking," Claveau said. "Her next goal is living back in her own house with her seven-year-old daughter, which is something she will achieve. She's an inspiration and has worked very hard over the last couple of years."

Doyle said she would not have been able to recover without the support of her family. Her mother and father stayed in Portland and wouldn't leave her side. Her dad, Leon, took six months off from his job at Bath Iron Works.

While she was in a coma, her grandmother, Phyllis Doyle, of Gardiner, cared for her daughter, Tiffany, a second-grader at Chelsea Elementary School. Her sister, Jennifer Doyle, of Chelsea, helped with Tiffany and so did the child's father, Christopher McGuire, of Augusta. Doyle said she wants another kidney transplant, but her lungs are still not at 100 percent. And because her case is so unusual, doctors can't say if she would be a good candidate for another transplant.

"I ask them how long before I can have a transplant, but there's nothing in the textbooks about what I have lived through and the progress I've made," she said. "Every step of the way, they have told me you aren't ever going to do any better. That's all I heard for two years and every time I got better. You'd think they'd stop saying it to me." ~ **Mechele Cooper, *Kennebec Journal***

June 28, 1999: I have recently survived Legionnaires' and I was upset [by] the fact that there is such little public awareness as to its cause. I had a very scary hospital course and almost died. I am an RN and was caught by surprise nonetheless with the first symptom which was basically a painful neck and inability to move my head to the right without pain. I therefore dismissed that symptom since I was busy at work until it was too late. I have since been through a ventilator, dialysis, stomach feedings, a tracheotomy, and a cardiac catheterization. I'm presently recuperating but very angry [about] the lack of information and precautions, and that this is not a matter of public awareness. I feel I have just paid a very high price for my ignorance. Please RSVP if there's anything I can do to help spread information. Thank You.

More information given on October 31, 2001: My case was confirmed via sputum and urinary [tests] as far as I can remember.

… I had no energy and my husband was complaining that I was becoming disoriented but even then I thought it was possibly a late flu.

However my temperature was 104°F and I finally went to the doctor. At that point I could barely walk. He diagnosed me with pneumonia and put me on Zithromax. Being a nurse, I was determined to give the antibiotic three days. On the third night, I could feel my lungs collapsing and we called an ambulance. I could no longer walk. I was admitted and apparently had a respiratory arrest and was intubated. Things went from bad to worse as they waited for the cultures. When it was confirmed as Legionnaires', the docs started three antibiotics and I was sent to the ER for a tracheotomy for the respirator. I was no longer awake for any of this. I then went to the OR again for a stomach tube so they could feed me. The Legionnaires' hit my heart next and it was feared than I was going into congestive heart failure, and my pancreas was unable to produce insulin so they began insulin and morphine drips. My husband said that at one point I had 15 bags going into me and he was unable to get to my side. My kidneys then went and I was in renal failure and needed dialysis. My blood pressure was almost nonexistent ... I had about 11-15 specialists on my case and over 35 X-rays. I woke up after the dialysis was over and they weaned me off an ativan drip, at which point, if I could have communicated or moved anything on my body, I would have escaped from the nightmare. I had to have speech therapy and everyone was nervous that I might have suffered anoxia and if so I would [not] remember how to talk, spell, etc. I was scared, too, and initially spelled "cat" k-a-t. I was completely helpless.

... The public health dept could not find any Legionnaires' where I worked. They only cultured the public drinking water. Why? If they're the experts, why didn't they culture anything else?

It wasn't until I read about Legionnaires' that I remembered going to the dentist and also about that blast of air from the vents outside where I worked that had thrown me against the wall. I was completely distressed and oh so incredibly furious to find out that one could also get it from ... cruise ships, dentists, food mists in supermarkets, and spas, as well as the usual places already known like stagnant water around construction sites.

I was laid up for another three months trying to rehab myself because I refused to go to a nursing home or rehab hospital and had to learn how to write again.

My husband took care of the tracheotomy and stomach dressings, as well as bathed me. I was unable to care for myself all because it hadn't even occurred to me that I had been exposed to something so deadly and so accidentally.
I will never forget the suffering of both me and my family and the fear as to where this came from and whether to resume my normal life when I was able. I

would like this condition to be as public as AIDS, TB, Hepatitis, and Anthrax. Please let me know if there's anything I can do. I wouldn't wish this syndrome on my worst enemy. ~ **A. F.**

I was recently diagnosed with Legionnaires' disease. I am a scrub nurse in a hospital OR. I went to my doctor and requested to be tested for Legionnaires' because several coworkers were sick with similar symptoms and one of my coworkers mentioned LD. He was reluctant to test me. I insisted, and thank God I did. When I first got sick, I thought pneumonia. Of course nurses aren't allowed to get ill so I just kept muddling through until I could no longer swallow my own sputum or take a breath without pain. If it weren't for a co-worker insisting I be persistent with my physician, I would never have known that I had LD, and could've died. I want to thank you for this website and all the abundance of information you supply. I may be a nurse but had never encountered LD and was not aware of all the symptoms or the treatment or the severity. ~ **W. W., September 2001**

October 2003: I'm in Cranbrook, BC and I contracted Legionnaires' disease.

The Public Health people told me I probably contracted it where I worked. They also told me they didn't have the manpower to investigate further.

I felt ill on July 4th but still went ahead with plans to visit Radium Hot Springs here in BC Canada. After visiting the pools (both the public and the small hot pool), the next morning I was extremely worse and we left early to head back to Cranbrook to the hospital.

The doctor there said I was fine, gave me a new inhaler, and sent me on my way. Two days later, even worse, I went in and saw my family doctor. She said the same thing.

On Friday July 11th, I entered my doctor's office in tears. She sent me for an X-ray at the hospital and I was told immediately by the X-ray tech to have a seat [because] I wasn't going anywhere.

I remember absolutely nothing from this moment on ... not being admitted, being restrained by security because I wanted to go home, hitting the nurse, or being air-lifted by a helicopter on life support to Calgary Foothills Hospital two days later (Sunday).

I remember nothing for 10 days after this. I was sent back to Cranbrook Hospital on July 23rd. I got my breathing and asthma sort of under control, and I signed myself out of the hospital on the 27th. (I'm a single mom and needed to be at home.)

I tried to go back to work around mid-September but couldn't do it ... ended up home in tears because I'd lose my breath just trying to talk to customers. And the lack of energy is crazy! I'd nap every few hours ... sometimes 18 hours per day.

I started working two days a week on October 1st with permission from my doctor. The first few weeks were tough ... my poor muscles were so sore, felt like I was gonna die when I got home.

I'm not doing too well. I have no fingernails left and all I want to do is eat. Every muscle in my body is aching and wakes me up during the night. I guess these are the "down" days I've been told will happen for 1-2 years following recovery.

Update in February 2010: It's been 6.5 years now and I still struggle with long-term memory loss. It took over a year before I was able to work again. I still have a scar on my chest from where they punched a big needle to try and resuscitate me on the helicopter on our way to Foothills Hospital in Calgary. The reports say I was completely dependent on life support to keep me breathing ... without it, I would have died.

Luckily for me, there'd been a recent case in Calgary and the doctor on call that night at Foothills was on the ball enough to test me for LD. I spent the next three months in and out of hospitals.

There are still memories from the past that are gone. I have "black holes" where the memories should be. Family members talk about my Grandfather's funeral and I don't even remember him dying or me being present during that time. I've lost most of my memories of my youngest daughter's life from ages 1-6 ... they just vanished.

It was the worst experience of my life and an eye-opener for me. From that moment, I changed my life. I realized I had to focus my entire energies on being healthy for my children and my entire outlook on life changed. I appreciate the small things more; I live every day like it's my last and I say "I love you" to my family members and close friends every single chance I get. ~ **D. D., BC, Canada**

I have recently been diagnosed with Legionnaires' disease. My doctor says he doesn't need to report it. He also admits he doesn't know much about it. I have been on three different antibiotics.

I have been sick for about three weeks now and have lost time from work. When can I go back to work? How long should I stay on the antibiotic?

Should I report my disease to the CDC? I'd like to know where I contracted it. I went on vacation to Maui (I live in California); could it have been the hotel spa, pool, shower, or air-conditioning system? Could I have gotten it on the airplane ride home? Should I alert the hotel or the airlines? I don't want anyone else to get the disease, if possible. ~ **Kathleen, Concord, CA, September 20, 2003**

My husband contracted Legionnaires' in May of this year. He spent 10 days in the intensive care unit of our local hospital. Upon release, he was given oxygen tanks and several meds and was told to be on bed rest for at least two weeks. The county health department took samples at his workplace—which happens to be a major hotel chain—and also at a hotel we stayed at for vacation the weekend prior to his illness.

My husband did not ask to contract Legionnaires'. He did not look to get this horrible sickness, however his employer is treating him as if he sought out the germ and inhaled it purposely. I do not feel that our American workplace understands, or cares to take the time to understand, what Legionnaires' is and how it affects the human body. ~ **Rose, July 2006**

November 2003: My ex-uncle-in-law is dying from Legionnaires' disease. Why can't they give him a lung transplant? They're so desperate that he was put in a coma and given steroids. They say he would die if they try to open his chest. Why? He was on the road to recovery and all of a sudden turned bad.

Update in March 2004: I am excited to tell you that my ex-uncle-in-law beat the odds. He's home and has rehab several times a week. Against all odds and the doctors' beliefs, he made it. From what I heard, the source of contamination was found to be in one of the water fountains in a common area. ~ **M. L., Boston, MA**

My wife was a patient in [hospital name] in March of 2001 recovering from a brain aneurysm operation and was doing well. About seven to eight days after her clip was performed, she developed pneumonia. Within two days, she was in a coma. After several days of testing, it was discovered that she had Legionnaires' disease. The poor thing was in a coma for the better part of two months.

The hospital has never taken any responsibility for the cause of the disease.

Can you advise me if there is any type of lung infection or other problems with the lungs with Legionnaires' survivors? We are looking hard for answers. ~ **T. B., February 2004**

My next door neighbor was diagnosed officially by the Mayo Clinic as having Legionnaire's disease. I do not think they found out how he got it. He started being very sick for about a week at home and then finally went to the ER unable to breath very well. He woke up from a coma six days later. He had a tracheotomy to save his life in the ER and was very sedated in intensive care thereafter and very sick. Was weeks in the hospital and very weak for more weeks at home. The doctors have told him it will be at least a year until he's normal.
~ **Judy A. Collins**

My 19-year-old son died on June 26, 2005 at [hospital name] Medical Center. He was admitted to a positive pressure isolation room on April 13, 2005 for a stem cell transplant for his leukemia. He began having pneumonia symptoms in mid-May that was thought to be fungal, although bronchial cultures never came back positive. He was treated with Ampho-B, both aerosol and I.V., even though cultures came back positive for gram negative bacteria. He was in remission and recovering his cell count (from his identical twin donor) when he was admitted to ICU and put on a respirator. At that time, Legionella was suspected and tested for in his urine and in another bronchial lavage. The Ampho-B was stopped and treatment for the Legionella began. He died 12 days later in ICU from respiratory and organ failure in spite of the fact that the right lung had improved. The Ampho-B and the delay in diagnosis had already done too much damage.

At my son's memorial service, his stem-cell doctor commented to me that [hospital name] "couldn't even keep their vents clean." The hospital did not report my son's Legionnaires' disease to the county health department until July 13 and I do not know what kind of testing they did on their own or if the health department responded.

There was another pediatric patient one room away from my son that was having similar symptoms who disappeared one night shortly before my son was sent to ICU. I don't know what happened to her.
~ **Deanne McDonald, Murrieta, CA, July 29, 2005**

I am a kind of healthy 26-year-old who contracted LD in May 2003 ... from a five-star spa whilst on holiday. Due to the incubation period, I didn't get ill until I arrived back in England. I was in the hospital for four days before they tested me and diagnosed LD.

It affected my family hugely, especially my mother—she came to the hospital every day to wash and dress me! As I'm sure you can imagine, this was very degrading for me but exactly what mothers do, and I couldn't thank her enough. I was in there for 14 days and had to take approximately three months off of work.

After a long recovery, I have been feeling relatively better for a long time. But since I have had LD, I seem to be getting ill all the time … if it isn't ear infections, it's the flu or viruses and it always seems to take me ages to recover compared to a "normal person."

I just wonder if having LD could have affected my immune system and made me susceptible to infection. ~ **Sally Goulden, Potters Bar, Hertfordshire**

I contracted the disease last year and spent some six weeks in intensive care and a renal unit. I was taken in unconscious and am glad to say have made a full recovery. I had a temporary kidney failure but that was resolved by treatment. I was told that if I had not been a tough old bird (I'm 73), I would not have survived. So there is hope after Legionnaires'. ~ **Mike Clinch, London, January 2006**

I contracted Legionnaires' in December 2005, spending just under 30 days in the ICU on life support. Complications included meningitis and double pneumonia. After lots of home therapy, I continue to have what doctors claim to be nerve distortion in my upper right shoulder. This continues to be very frustrating and extremely painful. I also now (rarely before) suffer from intense light and sound sensitive migraines. Could this be a side effect? ~ **T. F., January 2007**

I have just returned home from attending the funeral of my sister's father-in-law. The family got a call today that the cause of death was Legionnaires' disease. The deceased was a diabetic and he also had cystic fibrosis. Seventy-four years old. Non-smoker. We are guessing that he contracted it while at a convention in Georgia.
~ **George Fordham, Clarksburg, WV, June 2007**

My 64-year-old father was recently diagnosed as having Legionnaires' disease. He, my mother, my three-year-old son, and I were in Niagara Falls, Canada last week. I suspect that he was infected through the hotel's air-conditioning system. Is there any way to request testing on their cooling system to confirm or deny that it is where he contracted this disease? He is currently in the hospital and more than likely will not be able to return to work for quite a while. We went on this vacation to enjoy my son seeing Niagara Falls for the first time. Now it has turned into a nightmare both physically and financially for my parents. I truly believe that someone needs to be held responsible for what happened to my father ... that someone should be held responsible for improper maintenance on equipment, especially [since it's a] place that is frequented by tourists. ~ **Kelly Fagan-Dyer, Washington, PA, September 2007**

My husband was in the hospital for 18 days and almost died. He was first told he had pneumonia and then got ARDS [Acute Respiratory Distress Syndrome] and had to be put on a ventilator for 12 days. It was at that time I was told he had Legionnaires' disease. He is a sheet metal worker and prior to getting [sick] was working on the same jobsite for a long time. One week before he started showing symptoms, he had been sent to two different job sites. I know he got this from work. Within two weeks prior to getting sick, he didn't go anywhere but home and work. The insurance company does not want to test the jobsite [where] we think he got it. Any suggestions as far as what we could do? ~ **Erica, September 2007**

October 18, 2007: I was told two days ago by my doctor that I had Legionnaires' [based on] a blood test he did following about a month of coughing and fevers. I was given an antibiotic by the first doctor I saw and my second doctor seems to think nothing else needs to be done. I continue to have low fever and am coughing and very weak all the time. What else should I do? See another doctor? Also, after ten years, I finally got drawn for an elk tag in Arizona and am debating if I should try to go on the hunt this week.

After reading about what Legionnaires' is, I am more scared that maybe I should be doing something else to make sure I have defeated it. My body does not feel right and I am tired of being weak and coughing all the time. Can you give me any advice as to what else if anything I should be doing?

Update February 2010: I didn't go elk hunting or probably would not be here today.
This disease was the worst thing medically I have ever experienced and had I not been healthy when I got it, I would probably have died. I have not been in a spa since. I also stay out of hospitals and places with large

water evaporative devices if I can. ~ **Mark Fooks, Glendale, AZ**

September 10, 2008: My husband contracted Legionnaires' at [Name] University in [City], PA. He was so severe that he almost did not make it. He is permanently disabled and suffers from long-term sequelae from the Legionnaires' disease.

I wish that there would have been a policy for individuals and cooling towers. My husband's first symptom was a headache [and then] migraines, then joint pain (hips and shoulders). He continues to have these and there appears to be no relief despite multiple treatment modalities. His symptoms remain with periods of exacerbations. He now has COPD [Chronic Obstructive Pulmonary Disease] and scar tissue in his lungs that he did not have before and this resulted in his lung collapsing and double pneumonia nine months after he experienced the near fatal Legionella pneumonia. He also developed cardiomegaly with a new onset of hypertension. His short-term memory is also an issue. My husband has a team of doctors and we have been told that, although rare, these are a direct result of the Legionnaires'. These physicians have deemed my husband permanently disabled. [He was exposed] on 6/15/07, started to develop symptoms on 6/25/07, and was hospitalized on 7/1/07. Do you know of any treatments? We are at our wits' end.

Update, February 12, 2010: Larry [still] has headaches and migraines. His joint pain remains. He becomes short of breath and utilizes a nebulizer about four times a day.

He has been hospitalized seven times since the onset of
Legionnaires' in 2007. Prior to the Legionnaires', he was
a vibrant man. We have three small children that he used
to be able to keep up with—he is no longer able to do
this. We both know that he is lucky to be alive, but his
quality of life has drastically changed. It has placed a
huge strain on our family. ~ **Kristine Fierman,
Broomall, PA**

I am a 43-year-old single mom and was recently
blindsided by Legionnaires'. I went to my Urgent Care
clinic with what I thought was bronchitis after about five
days of a dry cough and then developed a fever. I was
diagnosed with pneumonia, admitted to the hospital, and
the next thing I knew I was waking up in ICU with a
breathing tube in my throat, only to find out I had been
in a COMA FOR 5 DAYS!!!

All I could think was "my poor family" (I have a 7-year-
old son and we live with my 81-year-old father). When I
was told I had Legionnaire's disease, I knew nothing
about the illness. I vaguely remembered the outbreak in
the 1970s but that's about it. My case is about as severe
as you could get and live through it. I was in a coma, on
a respirator, my kidneys failed, I needed continued
dialysis for days, and my other organs were failing. I
found out later that they finally brought my son to see
me on the fifth day and I woke up that night (I truly
believe he brought me back).

Does anyone actually know how the disease [is
contracted]? My family assumed it was an old window
air-conditioner in my room and removed it immediately.

Since I was the only case reported in my county, the health department won't come to the house to do an investigation.

Also, do you have to have prolonged exposure to *Legionella* bacteria or can you get sick from just one exposure? I've had so many complications since being released from the hospital. I had to have two more weeks of dialysis, then I developed a blood clot in my neck where my renal catheter had been and had to go on Warfarin and give myself Lovenox injections twice a day in my stomach (yuck!). And right now I think I have an infection in one of my many IV sites.

I am very interested in hearing other [LD] stories and information about long-term problems. My doctors just weren't that informative. ~ **Marcia B., Wisconsin, September 6, 2008**

I was just wondering if a public swimming pool could be the cause for Legionnaires' disease. My son has just been diagnosed with this, and shortly before this, he joined the swim team. He is a healthy, 12-year-old boy who doesn't get sick very often. Please let me know if this is possible because I don't know if I want to keep him on the swim team. Thanks so much. ~ **L. J., November 22, 2008**

I was just recently released from the hospital and nearly died from Legionnaires'. I have no idea how I got it. I live in Amherst, NH and work in Chelmsford, MA. The CDC was contacted but I've heard nothing from them and so far I haven't heard of any other cases in this area. We have bleached the water system here and have had samples tested which have all come back negative. Do you know how I can find out if there have been any other recent cases in New Hampshire? ~ **G. R., Amherst, NH, February 9, 2009**

July 28, 2009: I am 47 years old (male), do not smoke or drink, and was in healthy physical condition. I contracted the disease in February 2009 and was treated in the hospital one week later. The doctor that treated me in the ER had experience with LD 13 years prior and figured out what I had within one hour of my being admitted to the hospital.

My experience with LD in the hospital and recovery at home was the worst thing I have ever been through. After three weeks from the time they discovered the disease, the doctor told me the only way to get over the fatigue and shortness of breath was to exercise and walk. I started my rehab and after two months was back at work. My weight is back up (I lost 30 pounds) and I am feeling stronger than ever physically. However, after five months, I still have a major problem with short-term memory—I forget where I am going, or forget people's names even though I have known them for years.

Is there a vitamin that I can take? How long will this side effect last?
Please help. It seems like the long-term effects from LD are worse than the hospital experience.

Update February 15, 2010: It's been one year since this happened and the only problem I have left is the shortness of breath! The good news is the more I push myself, the better I feel. I think I will be fully recovered by this summer. It's a miracle! ~ **Steve Sederstrom**

I was on holiday in Cancun, Mexico last September. I traveled from the UK. I was particularly well and reasonably fit for my age (54). After a few days, at a reasonable hotel (four-star), I contracted an illness that I assumed was "heat stroke" and simply drank water and ate very little, resting in my room in the air-conditioning. On my return home, after an awful air trip and a 180-mile drive, I saw my general practitioner who fortunately recognized the symptoms as LD [and] sent me straight to a hospital. I was treated in special care with antibiotics, along with oxygen. After 10 days, I was sent home and regularly checked by my GP for a number of weeks. After 3-1/2 months, I returned to work on light duty. ~ **M. F., Devon, UK, July 31, 2009**

My husband tested positive for *Legionella* in 2008. He went through the antibiotics and they even gave him high doses of steroids. I am very concerned because he is still tired all the time. His concentration is not even close to what it used to be. He can't remember things from one day to the next. He writes just about everything down so he won't forget.

I am very concerned that the bacteria might have caused damage in the heart and brain while it was living inside him. Is it possible that the bacteria have done damage to other organs? ~ **A. T., August 2009**

My husband was a patient in a local hospital for treatment of a platelet disorder and developed Legionnaires' disease. He had his spleen removed and was on many immune suppressant medications including chemotherapy.

I noticed the ceiling tiles in his room were wet, not from a leaky roof, but probably the AC duct above the ceiling tile. Do you think that this may have caused this disease? I really want to narrow this down. I want to make sure he contacted it in the hospital, not at our home.

He spent a total of about 50 days in the hospital during a three-month period. ~ **C. F., Boonton, NJ, August 2000**

December 3, 2001: I survived a very severe case of *Legionella longbeachae* in May of 2000. The hospital teaching staff used my X-rays in their classes. [After my case,] they made it policy to test all pneumonia patients for both *Legionella pneumophila* and *Legionella longbeachae*.

I don't know all the technical details of my ordeal as I don't understand the medical notes. But I can tell you that I was the first case reported to have acquired this disease in the US from commercial potting soil. I almost died. The doctors had told my family that I would probably not live an additional hour. They were all amazed I lived. I wish I understood the notes and could tell you more. But I think the main thing is education to the medical staff. Too many doctors look only at the most common ailments and don't consider the less common diseases. Then someone dies and there is no alarm set off as to the cause of death.

Update February 16, 2010: My symptoms were like flu symptoms until I had a hard time breathing. The bacteria spread so rapidly in my lungs that the X-rays were taken every couple hours instead of two times a day. I also ended up with sepsis which I think means my body was infected throughout and went into shock. When the body went into shock, the blood vessels expanded and the blood was not being moved through them to the brain or various other parts of the body. The doctor could not get a blood pressure. They thought I was dead.

Except for severe nerve damage on my right foot and leg, I am doing very well. It has taken a long time to heal emotionally and physically. I had thought the nerve damage was because of neglect by the nursing staff, but I am more inclined to believe the damaged sciatic nerve was due to infection. I have not a clue for sure though. ~ **S. T., Renton, WA**

3. How to avoid Legionnaires' disease in public places

Sources of *Legionella* contamination

Cases of Legionnaires' have been linked to plumbing systems, cooling towers, respiratory care equipment, showers, faucets, whirlpool spas and baths, humidifiers, decorative fountains, and a grocery store mist machine.

Cooling towers

Cooling towers are used to cool water for air-conditioning or industrial equipment. Inside cooling towers, water cascading downward intersects air moved by large, powerful fans. Most of the water falls into a basin at the bottom of the cooling tower but some of it is blown into the air.

Cooling tower water is prone to *Legionella* contamination because of its temperature and exposure to airborne particles. Cooling towers have been implicated in many outbreaks on the theory that

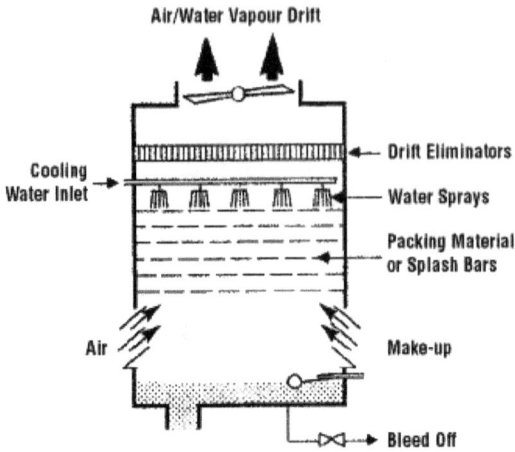

Cooling tower diagram. *Courtesy Canadian Centre for Occupational Health and Safety*

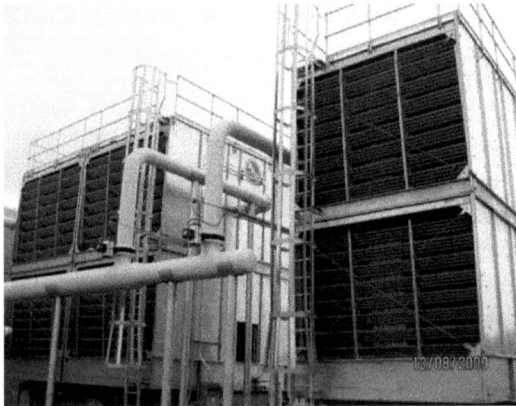

Cooling towers

Legionella-contaminated mist drifted from the tower to people inside a building through an outdoor air intake or through windows, or directly to people in the vicinity of the cooling tower.

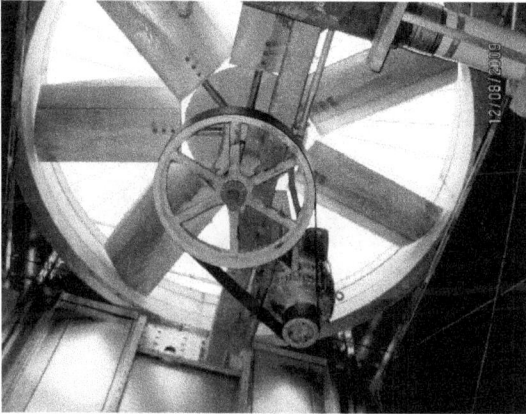

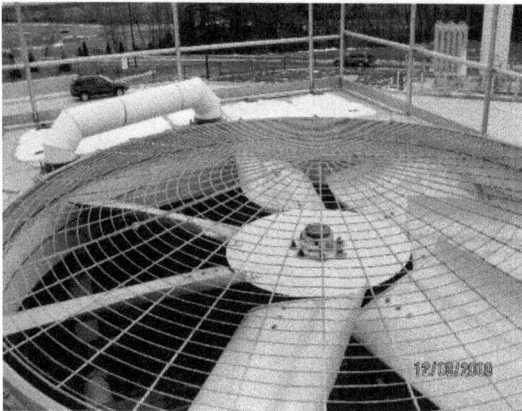

The large fan pulls air into the cooling tower and blows it outside.

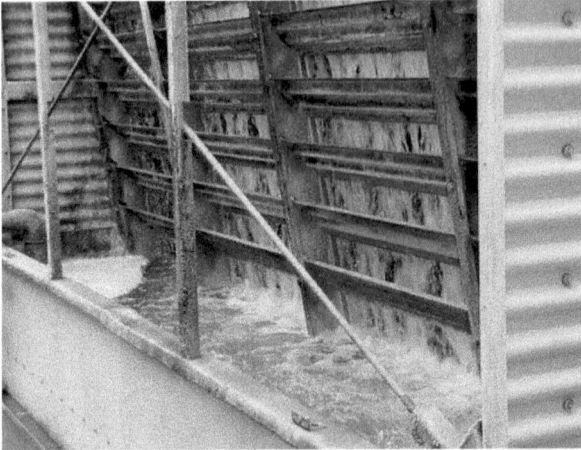

Water cascades through fins ("fill") and falls into the basin.

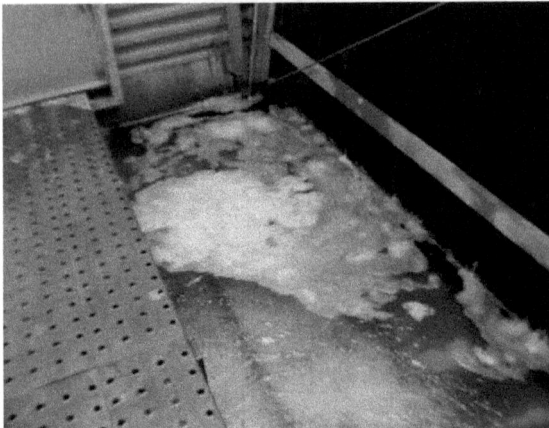

The basin collects water that cascades down from the top of the cooling tower.

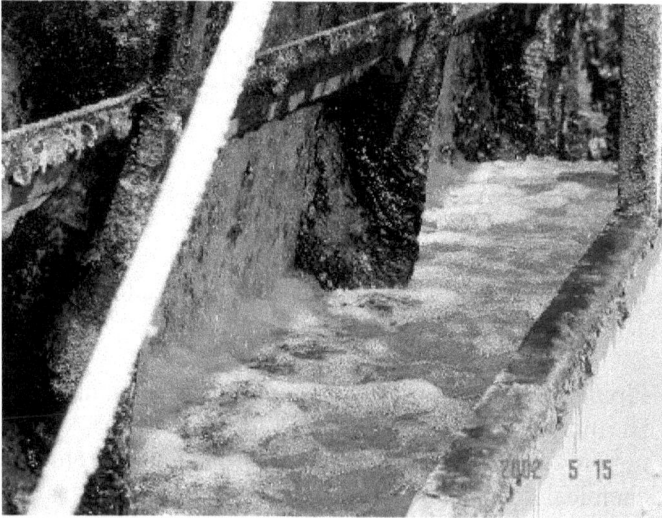

Cooling towers get dirty without proper cleaning and water treatment. The slime is thick on this one.

Plumbing systems

Plumbing systems have been implicated in many Legionnaires' outbreaks.

Although the US EPA has set forth a goal of zero *Legionella* in public water supplies, water companies do not have to test for *Legionella,* and the bacteria tests that the EPA does require (coliform tests) do not indicate the presence or absence of *Legionella.*

The EPA acknowledges that public water supplies typically contain *Legionella* bacteria at very low concentrations—lower than what can be detected by laboratories. But water is more prone to *Legionella* growth *after* it leaves the public water distribution system and enters a building's plumbing, where it finds warmer temperatures, stagnation, and smaller pipes, valves, and fittings.

Plumbing systems make a perfect habitat for *Legionella* bacteria. *Legionella* can flourish in a water heater, especially at the bottom, where the water is not as hot and where scale (hard water deposits) and sediment accumulate.

Piping presents a more complex problem than tanks. Biofilms that form on valves and fittings and pipe walls not only feed the bacteria but also protect them from chemical disinfectants. Biofilm is a slimy coating that is formed as microbes attach to underwater surfaces (the inside of a pipe).

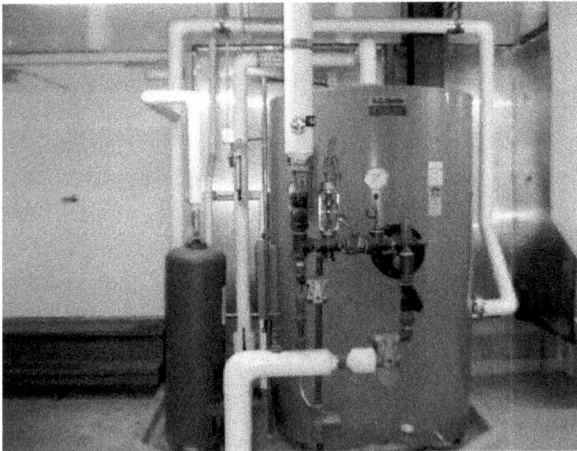

500-gallon tank for water heating and storage

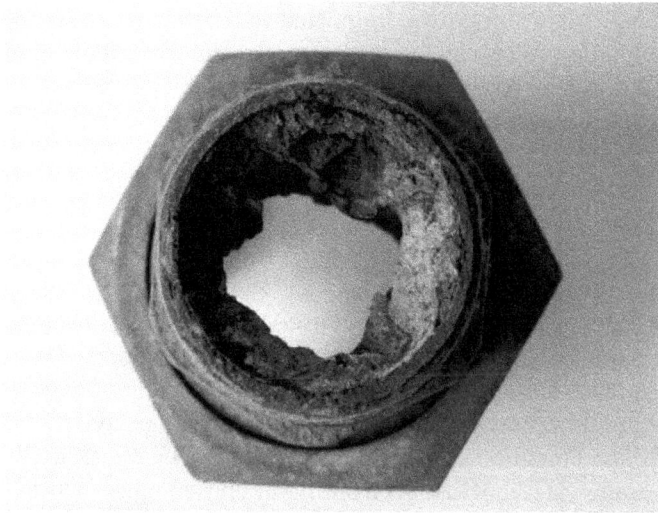

This pipe fitting is occluded by scale and other debris.

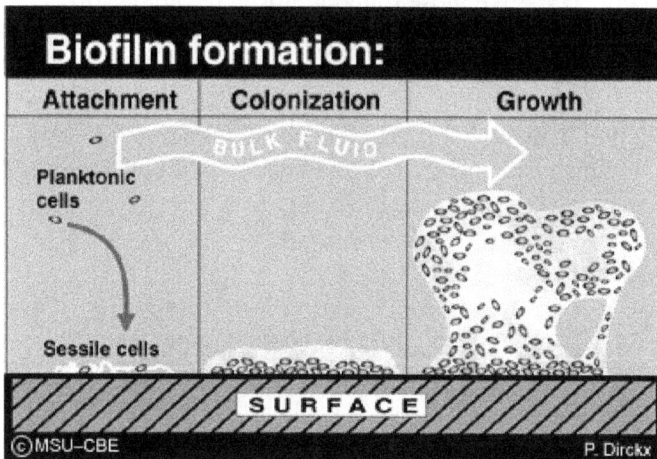

Picture courtesy Montana State Univ.

As the biofilm grows, fragments of it break off and flow into the water, delivering potentially high levels of *Legionella* to faucets, showers, and drinking fountains. Many outbreaks of Legionnaires' disease have been associated with construction projects and water main work because vibration or water pressure shock can loosen biofilm from piping.

Water that has become stagnant—whether because of system design or infrequent use—is another *Legionella* promoter in plumbing systems. Cases of Legionnaires' disease have been associated with the opening of new buildings or re-opening of idle building areas; under these conditions, *Legionella* bacteria can be released from water that had been sitting in unused pipes.

Large plumbing systems with complex piping networks—like those found in hospitals, hotels, office buildings, and large apartment buildings—are especially prone to *Legionella* growth. Home plumbing systems are not exempt, though. In fact, *Legionella* bacteria has been found in many home plumbing systems surveyed, some of which have been implicated in cases of Legionnaires' disease.

Whirlpool spas

Whirlpool spas (hot tubs) are another major source of Legionnaires' disease. Many people have contracted Legionnaires' disease after using hotel hot tubs. These cases often result in lawsuits, claiming the hotel inadequately maintained the hot tub. Data is not available to indicate the prevalence of Legionnaires' cases associated with home hot tubs.

Cooling towers, plumbing systems, and hot tubs are responsible for the vast majority of Legionnaires' disease cases. In hospitals, respiratory therapy equipment is another important source. Decorative fountains, humidifiers, and misters have also been implicated in Legionnaires' cases. Dental water lines have been strongly suspected as a cause of Legionnaires' disease but have not been implicated by a method that satisfies the scientific community.

Controversy over risk reduction strategies

The risk of Legionnaires' disease in building water systems can be greatly reduced by minimizing Legionella bacteria in them.

There are two basic public health approaches to Legionnaires' disease, **proactive** and **reactive**. In essence, a reactive strategy is to do little or nothing to rid water of *Legionella* until someone gets sick. One of the problems with this approach is that, as mentioned in Chapter 1, most cases of Legionnaires' disease go undetected, so a water system could cause a lot of illness and death before it is recognized as hazardous. A second problem is that even if a case is diagnosed and successfully treated, the survivor's life may still be significantly affected, as you saw by the survivors' stories in Chapter 2.

The proactive approach is to take reasonable steps to minimize *Legionella* bacteria in water systems even if no cases of Legionnaires' disease have been associated with that building. For most buildings, these preventive measures are just good maintenance and can be done at a reasonable cost.

A proactive risk reduction strategy is implemented in four basic steps:

1. Take *Legionella*-preventive measures in the design, construction, operation, and maintenance of water systems.

2. Test the water for *Legionella* to determine if the preventive measures are working.

3. If the test results are not acceptable, then correct the situation (e.g., with a disinfection system or filters).

4. Go back to number 1.

Many countries have guidelines that recommend—or laws that require—*Legionella* prevention measures. These nations include Australia, Belgium, Czech Republic, Denmark, France, Germany, Ireland, Italy, Japan, Latvia, Malta, the Netherlands, Norway, Portugal, Singapore, South Africa, Spain, Switzerland, United Kingdom, and the United States.

Some Australian states and European countries require *Legionella* preventive measures and water testing with strict regulations that can result in prison terms if violated. In the United States, there are a number of government and industry guide documents regarding *Legionella,* but no federal or state laws requiring preventive measures or water testing. Most states follow the recommendations of the Centers for Disease Control and Prevention, which does not require, or even encourage, water testing for *Legionella* in hospitals or hotels where numerous cases of Legionnaires' disease occur each year. Some people think the CDC approach is reasonable. Others think it's dangerously lax.

Understanding your risk

Most people who are exposed to *Legionella* bacteria will not contract Legionnaires' disease, so there is no reason to panic. A reasonable degree of precaution is prudent, though.

You can reduce your risk of Legionnaires' disease by:

a. Lowering your susceptibility to infection and

b. Avoiding exposure to *Legionella* bacteria.

Consider risk-reduction measures based on the cost and your susceptibility to *Legionella* infection. Some risk-reduction measures cost nothing and should be implemented out of good sense. Expensive measures could be a waste of money for healthy nonsmoking adults, who are at low risk of contracting Legionnaires' disease, but could save the lives of high-risk individuals.

A key way to lower your susceptibility to Legionella infection is to stop smoking. Among persons who are not immunocompromised, smoking is the number one factor in acquiring Legionnaires' disease. A study of 146 adults with Legionnaires' disease indicated that for those who smoked one pack of cigarettes a day, the risk of contracting the disease was 121% higher than for nonsmokers. For each additional pack of cigarettes smoked daily, the risk increased another 121%.

Reducing your risk in hospitals and nursing homes

In 1999, *CNN and Time,* a television newsmagazine on CNN, reported that "every year, thousands of patients contract [Legionnaires'] disease from contaminated hospital water systems." The show included an interview with Dr. Victor Yu, a Legionnaires' expert from the University of Pittsburgh. "These outbreaks—they're actually occurring all through the country every week," said Yu. "It's an explosive problem to realize that people are dying, to realize that the means are there for preventing all this from happening, and that those means are not being exercised."

You cannot tell if a health facility has *Legionella* bacteria in its plumbing system simply by looking around. Signs of poor maintenance do not guarantee that a building has unsafe levels of *Legionella,* and signs of good maintenance do not guarantee that a building is *Legionella*-safe. Only periodic testing of water samples for *Legionella* will indicate whether or not a system is contaminated.

As a patient, you cannot do anything about the condition of the water in a health facility—this is the responsibility of the facility management staff—but you can reduce your risk of exposure by doing the following.

a. Ask questions before admission. In nonemergency situations, you have time to gather information about a health facility *before* admission. If you don't like what you hear, you can take precautions or choose another facility.

Call the infection control department of the hospital, or the manager of the nursing home, and ask these questions:

- What types of tests are available for identifying Legionnaires' disease? [Many hospitals do not make *Legionella* tests available to physicians.]

- Are patients with atypical pneumonia routinely tested for Legionnaires' disease?

- Do you sample water for *Legionella* routinely? How often?

- Do you have a written management plan for waterborne pathogens?

- Is a disinfection system installed in the plumbing system for *Legionella* control? What type of disinfectant is used? [The answer should be chlorine, copper-silver ions, or chlorine dioxide. Water softening is not a disinfection system for *Legionella.*]

- How many hospital-acquired cases of Legionnaires' disease have been identified in your health facility in the last five years? Which water system (plumbing system; cooling tower) was identified as the source of *Legionella* contamination? What remedial action was taken?

Have you continued to do follow-up sampling to validate the effectiveness of the remedial action?

Don't be afraid to make the telephone call. You do not need to be a Legionnaires' expert to discuss the above—the technical details are not necessary. The answers provided will indicate whether the health facility staff understands Legionnaires' disease and its risks and whether they work to prevent infection by controlling *Legionella*.

b. If you are diagnosed with atypical pneumonia, tell your physician that you want to be tested for Legionella.

If you asked the above questions prior to admission, you will already know whether or not the hospital makes *Legionella* tests available to physicians.

c. If you require a respirator or nebulizer, inquire about the cleaning practices.

Only sterile water (not distilled, nonsterile water) should be used for filling and rinsing nebulization devices and other respiratory care equipment. Avoid using these devices entirely if they are not absolutely necessary to your care.

d. Request bottled drinking water (or bring your own). Although hot-water systems are generally more conducive to *Legionella* growth than are cold water systems, *Legionella* can grow in the cold water lines as well, especially in hot climates where the temperature of the cold water may exceed 24°C (75°F). You can reduce your risk of *Legionella* infection by drinking bottled water or boiled tap water and by limiting your use of ice in beverages.

High-risk patients should also avoid showers. Even the use of bathtubs and faucets presents a *Legionella* risk.

Reducing your risk in office buildings

Theoretically, office buildings should not pose as great a threat of *Legionella* contamination as do hotels and hospitals. Office workers generally do not shower, brush their teeth, or wash their faces at work, and they are presumed to be in generally good health. Nevertheless, office buildings have been implicated in outbreaks of Legionnaires' disease.

Large multistory office buildings present a greater risk than smaller buildings because the plumbing systems are larger and more complex, and cooling towers may be used for air-conditioning. However, as explained above for health facilities, you cannot visually assess the *Legionella* risk in a building. Even if you observe factors conducive to *Legionella* growth—an extensive plumbing system, old piping, hot-water temperatures below 50°C (122°F), poor maintenance—these conditions do not guarantee that the building has unsafe levels of *Legionella.* Likewise, once again, the absence of such factors does not guarantee that a building is *Legionella*-safe.

If you don't manage the building, there is little that you can do to affect the condition of the water. However, you can take steps to avoid exposure:

- High-risk individuals should consider using cold water instead of hot water for hand-washing. Cold water is less likely to be contaminated with *Legionella*.

- If an office or kitchenette sink has a small water heater under it, set the water heater at 60°C (140°F), **but be aware that scalding is a risk at this temperature. Do not set the temperature at 60°C (140°F) if the area is occupied by children or others who may open a hot water faucet unaware of the risk of scalding.** Drain and clean the water heater once a year to remove all sediment and scale.

- If a cooling tower or decorative fountain is located near the building, follow the suggestions below about those devices.

Reducing your risk in hotels

Many Legionnaires' outbreaks have been traced to hotels. As with health facilities and office buildings, you cannot tell by looking whether a hotel's water system is contaminated with *Legionella*. The following measures may help to minimize your exposure to *Legionella* in a hotel:

- The water flowing out of a faucet or shower during the first few seconds after the valve is opened is more likely to contain *Legionella* and other bacteria than is the water that comes out after one or two minutes of flow—especially if the tap has not been used for a day or longer (e.g., if the room has been vacant). When you get to your hotel room, let hot water run from the faucet and shower for two or three minutes, then let cold water run for two or three minutes. Stay out of the bathroom while the water is running.

Consider taking a bath instead of a shower, particularly if you are at a relatively high risk of acquiring Legionnaires' disease.

- If a cooling tower or decorative fountain is located near the building, follow the suggestions below about those devices.

- Do not use the hot tub unless you're sure it has been properly maintained and treated, which you are unlikely to find out merely by asking the hotel personnel. Do not use it at all if you are at high risk of contracting Legionnaires' disease. *More about hot tubs in the next section.*

Reducing your risk from various types of equipment

Any device that can emit airborne water droplets should be considered a potential threat. Examples of potential hazards to avoid include misters, cooling towers, decorative fountains, and whirlpool spas and bathtubs.

Misters for comfort

In many arid cities and summertime amusement parks, misters line sidewalks and other public places to provide cooling. The temperature of the water that supplies the misters is likely to be in the *Legionella* growth range.

61

Although no published report has attributed a case of Legionnaires' disease to these misters, you should be cautious of these devices since they meet conditions conducive to *Legionella* infections. This includes the water being warm, stagnation, small pipe sizes, and the release of small water droplets.

Misters for food and plants

In 1989, an outbreak of Legionnaires' disease in Bogalusa, LA (USA) was traced by investigators to a grocery store mist machine. Thirty-three persons were hospitalized. The mist machine was an ultrasonic humidifier with a tank that contained relatively stagnant water. Lighting located beneath the humidifier may have warmed the tank water to temperatures conducive to *Legionella* growth. Ultrasonic humidifiers must be kept clean to prevent the growth of *Legionella* and other bacteria.

In 2000, a food display humidifier located in the dining area of a hotel in South Wales (UK) was blamed for five cases of Legionnaires' disease. Two individuals died of the disease. The strain of *Legionella pneumophila* found in the two patients who died was indistinguishable from isolates found in the humidifier. The humidifier was used to produce mist over food in a refrigerated display unit. Investigators found that the humidifier's antibacterial filters were missing and its ultraviolet lamp did not work.

Ultrasonic mist machines are uncommon in grocery stores. Most stores pipe water directly to spray nozzles, eliminating the water tank. Droplets produced by the spray nozzles are generally larger than those produced by ultrasonic machines and are thus less likely to be inhaled.

Cooling towers

Cooling towers are supposed to be maintained and treated to minimize the growth of bacteria. Many are not, however, and even well-maintained towers have been contaminated with *Legionella* at various times.

Cooling towers should be located as far as reasonably possible from operable windows, intake grilles through which outdoor air is brought into the building's ventilation system, parking lots, roads and driveways, sidewalks, and outdoor areas frequented by people. A minimum of 10 meters (33 feet) has been suggested, but 30 meters (100 feet) or farther is much safer.

You should attempt to stay at least 30 meters (100 feet) away from cooling towers. Wind can carry *Legionella* much greater distances, so the farther, the better.

If a cooling tower is located near the building in which you live or work, consider keeping your window closed, especially if the tower is within 10 meters (33 feet). Also, ask the building owner to relocate the outdoor air-intake for your building if it is within 10 meters (33 feet) of a cooling tower.

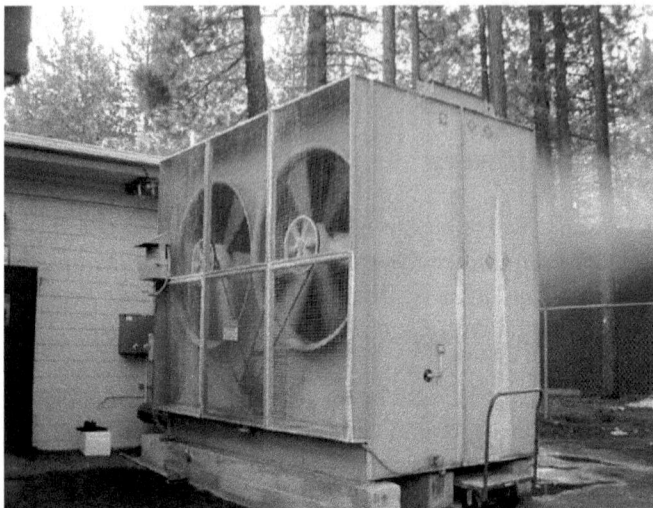

This small cooling tower is located at ground level close to a building. On the other side of the fence is a campground. You can see the mist discharged out of the back.

Decorative fountains

Decorative fountains have caused Legionnaires' disease. The fountains usually include a pump that sprays water, creating a mist that can be inhaled by people sitting around the fountain or walking by it.

You should be especially cautious if the bottom or sides of the fountain are covered with a greenish slime (algae), or if the water appears dirty.

The water in decorative fountains should be treated for the control of *Legionella* and other bacteria, and the fountains should be regularly cleaned, but many are inadequately maintained.

The risk of inhaling water droplets emitted by a fountain depends in part on the distance from the fountain to a person, the height and breadth of the spray, and the spray droplet size.

Look for factors that could promote bacteria growth. Submerged lighting could warm the water to temperatures more conducive to bacteria growth. Algae, and debris such as leaves, also promote bacteria growth. If the water appears dirty, be especially cautious.

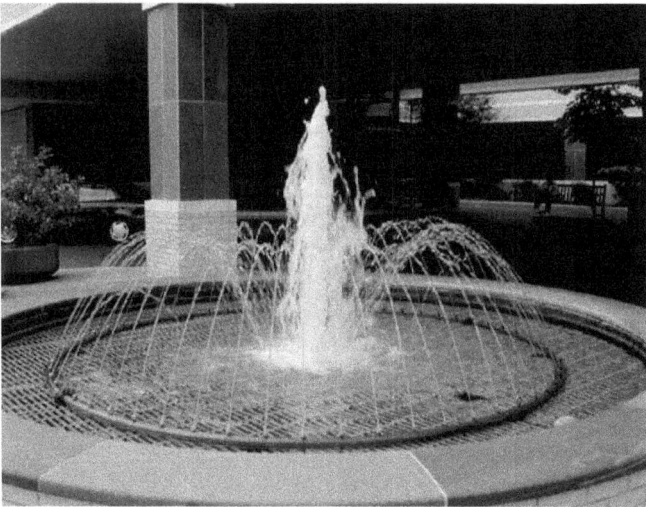

Given the height of the spray, water droplets or mist emitted from this fountain are likely to reach the breathing zone of people sitting on the benches around it.

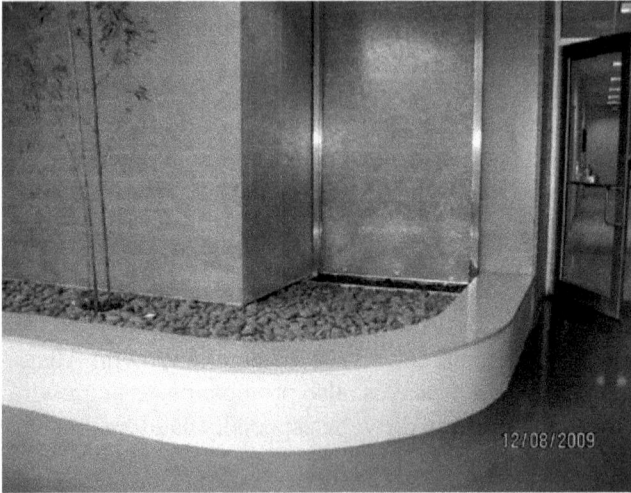

Water walls (where water flows down the wall) appear to emit little mist and for only a short distance but one was implicated in eight Legionnaires' cases in March 2010.

Whirlpool spas and bathtubs

Whirlpool spas (spas) are much the same as hot tubs except that spas are formed of plastic, concrete, or metal, while hot tubs are constructed with wood. In addition, spas are generally equipped with air jets, but many hot tubs are not. *For the purposes of this book, whirlpool spas, spas, and hot tubs are the same.*

Spas and hot tubs are not the same as whirlpool bathtubs. Spas and hot tubs are used for recreation rather than for bathing. Many spas are located outdoors. They are not drained after each use. Most have heaters. The water is treated and filtered.

Whirlpool bathtubs, however, are different. They are essentially bathtubs with water jets. Most are located in bathrooms. They are drained after each use. Most units do not have heaters, and the water is not treated with chemicals.

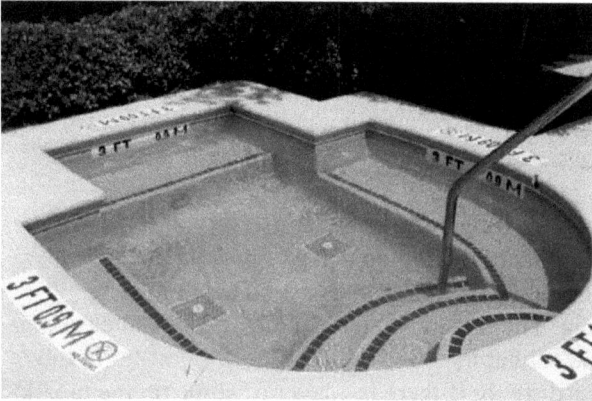

Whirlpool spa (hot tub)

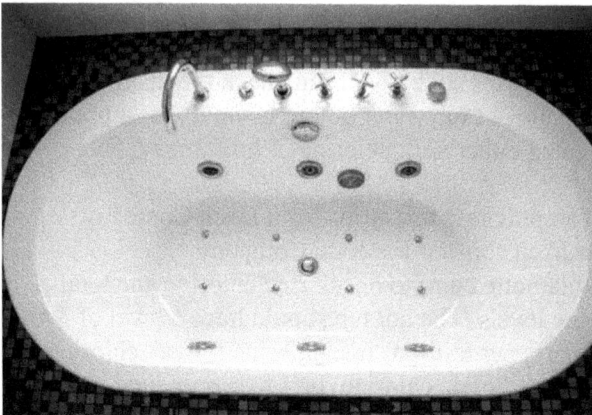

Whirlpool bathtub © Richliy, Dreamstime.com

Both types—hot tubs and whirlpool bathtubs—can provide a fertile breeding ground for many microbes, including *Legionella* bacteria. Hot tubs in hotels have been implicated in a number of Legionnaires' outbreaks. In 1994, 16 confirmed and 34 probable cases of Legionnaires' disease were traced to a whirlpool spa on a cruise ship.

If you have access to a public hot tub (at your exercise club), ask about the cleaning and maintenance practices before deciding whether to use it.

If you're visiting a facility (a cruise ship or hotel), you can do little to determine whether the spa or bath is contaminated with *Legionella.* You cannot tell by looking. The tub and water can look clean and clear and still be contaminated with bacteria. If the water or tub appear dirty, or if there is a layer of slime on the tub, do not use it. If the water and tub look clean, realize that you assume a degree of risk in using it.

If you travel frequently and like to use hot tubs, pack some test strips so that you can check the disinfectant level of the hot tub water before using it. Most hot tubs are treated either with chlorine or bromine.

You can purchase test strips from Hach Company (www.hach.com) or LaMotte Company (www.lamotte.com) to check free chlorine and total bromine levels. The hot tub should have a level of 3 to 5 ppm (parts per million) free chlorine ("free" chlorine as opposed to "total" chlorine) or 4 to 6 ppm total bromine. (Parts per million is sometimes expressed as milligrams per liter.) The swimming pool should have either 2 to 4 ppm free chlorine or 4 to 6 ppm total bromine.

If you own or operate a spa or whirlpool bathtub, read *Spas, Hot Tubs, and Whirlpool Bathtubs: A Guide for Disease Prevention* for guidance on water treatment, maintenance, and water testing (available at www.hcinfo.com).

High-risk individuals should not use a whirlpool spa or bath unless they know it is properly treated and cleaned and they have been cleared by their physician to use it.

You don't have to get in to get sick.

Studies of Legionnaires' outbreaks have shown that individuals can contract the disease, not only while using a whirlpool spa, but by spending time around one, or even walking in its vicinity. Data collected by investigators of a 2003 outbreak indicated that *Legionella* bacteria transmitted from a whirlpool spa may have infected people who were a significant distance from it.

In late February to early March of 1999, 242 people who visited a large flower show near Amsterdam (the Netherlands) became ill, and 28 died. Seemingly healthy people were among the victims. Legionnaires' disease was confirmed or considered probable in 192 of the cases and 21 of the deaths. *Legionella* bacteria were found in a spa that was on display at the show. The strain of *Legionella* found in the spa was identical to that found in some of the patients.

In November 1999, an outbreak of Legionnaires' disease was traced to a trade fair in the northern Belgian town of Kapellen. At least 80 persons developed symptoms similar to those caused by Legionnaires' disease. Positive urine tests confirmed Legionnaires' in 13 of the 80, and 4 of those 13 died. The World Health Organization reported that data from the initial investigation implicated working whirlpool baths exhibited at the show as the most likely source of infection.

A whirlpool spa display at a retail store in Virginia (USA) was blamed for 14 cases of Legionnaires' disease in 1996, including two deaths.

You should stay away from working (water filled) whirlpool spas or baths on display at stores or trade shows unless you know the spa or bath is being chemically treated to kill bacteria.

Windshield washing systems

The Health Protection Agency in the United Kingdom conducted a study to determine why professional drivers were five times as likely to acquire Legionnaires' disease as the general population in England and Wales. After finding that most of the drivers who contracted the disease drove cars that did not have chemically treated windshield washer fluid, the researchers concluded that the chemicals in screenwash kill *Legionella* bacteria that may otherwise thrive in stagnant washer water and therefore advised using screenwash instead of untreated water. They later ran tests and found *Legionella* in one in five cars that did not have screenwash, but in zero cars that did.

Reducing your risk in your job

If you work on or around cooling towers

Water treatment technicians and cooling tower maintenance workers probably have higher than normal antibodies against *Legionella* but can still be infected by bacteria emitted from cooling towers.

Although visibly dirty cooling towers are more likely than visibly clean ones to have high levels of *Legionella,* cooling towers that appear clean can be contaminated. Cooling tower workers should protect themselves by wearing a respirator while working around the tower. A high-efficiency respirator will block some but not all *Legionella* organisms.

If you work on the same tower periodically, the best way to protect yourself is to ensure that the tower is properly maintained to minimize *Legionella* growth.

If you work in a manufacturing facility

Water used in manufacturing can present a *Legionella* risk to workers.

For example, *Legionella* has been found in water used to cool molds in plastics forming-equipment. When workers change the molds or clean them with compressed air, water droplets can be sprayed into the air and inhaled.

In 1988, a fatal case of Legionnaires' disease was reported in an employee of a plastic injection molding plant. Investigators found high concentrations of *Legionella* bacteria (3,000 cfu/ml) in samples collected from the chilled water used to cool the molds.

High concentrations of *Legionella* were found in the chilled water used to cool metal molds and process equipment at another plastic injection molding facility (Cincinnati, OH, USA) where workers showed symptoms of Legionnaires' disease. The OSHA investigators reported that the chilled water systems were not treated with chemicals.

Subsequent to OSHA's investigation of the Cincinnati plant, an outbreak of Legionnaires' disease occurred among employees of a plastic injection molding facility in Baltimore, MD (USA). Legionnaires' disease was confirmed in five workers and suspected in three others. One of the workers died.

In December 1998, OSHA issued a Hazard Information Bulletin titled "Legionnaires' Disease Risk for Workers in the Plastic Injection Molding Industry." The alert is posted at www.osha.gov/dts/hib/hib_data/hib19981209.html.

If you work at a facility that uses water as part of manufacturing, check to confirm whether appropriate steps have been taken to minimize the growth of *Legionella* bacteria, particularly if water droplets can be released into the air.

If you work in a large building

Plumbing systems in houses and small commercial buildings can harbor *Legionella,* but *large plumbing systems are especially prone to bacteria growth.* Workers in hospitals, hotels, and office buildings have contracted Legionnaires' disease. *Smokers and individuals with compromised immune systems are at a higher risk.* (See the sections above about hospitals, hotels, and office buildings.)

If you work in such a building, ask about the waterborne pathogens management plan for the building.

Reducing your risk at the dentist

Lines carrying water to handheld dental devices are small in diameter, usually plastic, and sometimes even warm, making them conducive to biofilm development and growth of bacteria, including *Legionella.* As pieces of biofilm break loose from the inside of the tubing, potentially high doses of bacteria are released into the water. Once the bacteria reach the high-speed handheld dental devices, they are efficiently transmitted directly into the patient's mouth.

Ask your dentist what steps he or she takes to minimize harmful bacteria in water lines. More information about dental water line contamination is available at www.hcinfo.com.

4. How to avoid the disease at home

In a 1980s survey, mostly of apartments in a large building (87 apartment units and eight houses) in the Chicago area, *Legionella* was found in 30 of 95 residences (32%). In various surveys, *Legionella* has been found in single-family houses and duplexes, but, as expected, at a lower prevalence tan in large buildings (see table).

Legionella Surveys of Single-Family Houses and Duplexes

Area	Homes Surveyed	Homes with *Legionella*
Pittsburgh (USA)	55	6 (11%)
Quebec City (Canada)	54	11 (20%)
Germany, Netherlands, Austria	63	5 (8%)
Pittsburgh	218	14 (6.4%)
Quebec City	211	69 (33%)

People have contracted Legionnaires' disease from the water in their homes but having *Legionella* in your home plumbing does *not* mean you will get sick. None of the people who lived in the 30 Chicago residences (see first paragraph) or 14 Pittsburgh homes (see table) in which *Legionella* was found contracted Legionnaires' disease during the study period. If you are a nonsmoker in generally good health, your risk of contracting Legionnaires' disease at home is probably low unless the Legionella levels are high.

Nevertheless, everyone should consider taking risk reduction measures that cost little or nothing. The more costly measures probably do not make sense for young and healthy nonsmokers but may be prudent for immunocompromised persons.

Bear in mind that the following strategies are specifically for home plumbing systems. Steps that minimize *Legionella* bacteria in homes (small plumbing systems) may not be effective in large buildings.

Setting your water heater temperature

Set your water heater high enough to deliver 60°C (140°F) water to all taps but be aware that scalding is a risk at this temperature. **Do not use a high temperature setting if the house is occupied by children or others who may open a hot water faucet unaware of the risk of scalding.**

Legionella bacteria will die within about 32 minutes in a pot of water at 60°C (140°F) but they can survive these temperatures in some large, complex piping networks.

Keeping water at 60°C (140°F) will not always control *Legionella* in large buildings but has been effective in single-family residences. Water temperature was found to be a significant factor in at least four residential *Legionella* studies. In the Chicago study discussed above, all 30 samples in which *Legionella* was found were collected from water systems at temperatures under 60°C (140°F).

To check your hot water temperatures, simply place a thermometer in the stream of water flowing from a faucet. Faucets farthest from the water heater generally have the lowest temperatures, so check those to ensure that the water temperature remains sufficiently high (at or near 60°C/140°F) as it travels through the system. Be sure to check faucets nearest to the water heater as well to make sure that the water is not too hot—temperatures should not exceed 62°C (144°F).

Use a waterproof thermometer with a probe that is made for liquids. A digital thermometer will be faster and easier to read. In the United States, you can probably get one for under US$30 from Davis Instruments (www.davis.com), Foster and Smith Aquatics (www.fosterandsmithaquatics.com), or Hach Company (www.hach.com).

Don't assume that raising your water heater setting will increase energy costs. It may not. Further research is needed to make reliable calculations, and even then, the temperature-cost relationship will vary from house to house.

How to perform a hot water flush

Consider monthly flushes with superheated water if you keep your hot water lower than 60°C (140°F). Even if you maintain a higher temperature setting, flushes can provide added disinfection.

To conduct the hot water flush procedure:

a. Turn the water heater to its hottest setting.

b. Flush every tap for at least 30 minutes with 70°C (158°F) water. If your water heater doesn't have the capacity to flush all taps simultaneously (most home water heaters don't), flush one or two taps at a time for 15 minutes, beginning with those closest to the water heater and ending with the farthest taps. For maximum protection, also run the dishwasher and washing machine on the hottest setting.

    If your piping is old or in poor condition, consult a plumber about potential damage that the flushing procedure may cause. You may need to heat the water to 60°C (140°F) instead of 70°C (158°F), or not conduct the procedure at all.

c. Lower your water heater temperature to a safe setting after the hot water flush is completed.

Take these important precautions during each heat flush. Be sure that:

- Only nonsmokers in generally good health do the water flushing.

- Run the faucets at low to medium flow (no splashing) to minimize the release of potentially contaminated water droplets into the air.

- Immunocompromised persons are not in the house.

- Children or other potential scald victims are not in the house.

- Every person in the house is aware of the scalding risk.

What to do after returning from a vacation

Stagnant water promotes *Legionella* growth.

If you have been gone for a week, run all hot and cold water outlets for at least two minutes and flush all toilets. Only nonsmokers in generally good health should do the flushing. Run the faucets at low to medium flow (no splashing).

If you have been away for more than a week, or if the home is occupied by immunocompromised persons, then consider performing a hot water flush (described above).

Before moving into a home

Before occupying a home that has been vacant for a week or longer, at a minimum perform a hot water flush (described above), run all cold water outlets for at least four minutes (including hose bibbs if the outdoor temperatures are above freezing), and flush all toilets.

The flushing should be performed only by nonsmokers in generally good health. Run the faucets at low to medium flow (no splashing).

If you are moving into a single family house that has been vacant for several weeks or more, then consider injecting chlorine into the hot and cold water piping for disinfection. If you are renting rather than buying, you will obviously need to get approval from your landlord.

A chlorination procedure can take between 3 and 24 hours, depending on the concentration of chlorine. You won't be able to use the heavily chlorinated water so plan to have the procedure performed while the house is still vacant (but ideally no more than three days before you move in) or while you will be away from home.

Details about chlorinating plumbing systems are purposely omitted here because you should not do it yourself. Hire a plumbing contractor or water treatment specialist who has expertise and significant experience in chlorinating plumbing systems. Before agreeing to the procedure, have the specialist examine your piping to determine that the chlorine will not cause leaks or other damage.

After the chlorination, flush the system until the chlorine concentrations are at the levels in the public water supply.

The level of precaution you take will depend on your health, budget, and the condition of the home. An immunocompromised person preparing to occupy a home that has been vacant for months should certainly consider having the plumbing system chlorinated. For a healthy 20-year-old nonsmoker moving into a home that's been vacant for two weeks, hot and cold water flushing should be more than adequate.

Guest baths

Tiefenbrunner's research group found that homes with low water consumption were more likely to have *Legionella*-contaminated plumbing systems. At least once a week, run cold and hot water at all infrequently used faucets and showers for at least two minutes at low to medium flow (no splashing), and flush infrequently used toilets. The flush should be performed only by nonsmokers in generally good health.

After minor plumbing work

A study of 146 adults showed a higher risk of contracting Legionnaires' disease shortly after home-plumbing alterations or repairs were made. Repair work can loosen biofilm from piping and fixtures, releasing high levels of *Legionella* bacteria into the water.

After plumbing repairs are made, a nonsmoker who is in generally good health should run hot and cold water for at least five minutes at taps in the vicinity of the repairs.

If the plumbing work is extensive or involves significant vibration of the piping, consider performing a hot water flush to further reduce the risk, especially if the home is occupied by immunocompromised persons.

If your water becomes discolored

Outbreaks of Legionnaires' disease have occurred after events (water main repairs) that let dirt into the water supply or dislodge Legionella-laden biofilm and sediment from piping, often resulting in brownish colored water. If the water flowing out of your household faucets becomes discolored, run all hot and cold water outlets for at least two minutes and flush all toilets.

If the home is occupied by immunocompromised persons, then consider also performing a hot water flush as described above.

Remember that only nonsmokers in generally good health should do the flushing, and at low to medium flow (no splashing).

Before you buy your next water heater

When you purchase a water heater, consider gas instead of electric. Studies indicate that homes with gas water heaters are less likely to have *Legionella* than homes with electric water heaters.

Of 211 homes surveyed in the Quebec City area, *Legionella* was found in none of the 33 houses with gas water heaters but in 69 (33%) of the 178 houses with electric water heaters. The Pittsburgh study of 55 homes also showed a significant association between electric water heaters and *Legionella*.

Of the residential surveys discussed at the beginning of this chapter, the lowest *Legionella* positivity (6.4%) was found in the 218 Pittsburgh homes, 207 of which had gas water heaters.

The burner in gas water heaters is below the water tank, so the bottom of the tank, where sediment accumulates, is more likely to be sufficiently hot to prevent *Legionella* growth. In contrast, most electric units have heating elements on the side of the tank so the sediment at the bottom is at a lower temperature that is more favorable for *Legionella*.

Although data is not available to prove it, tankless water heaters may be less prone than tank-type heaters to *Legionella* contamination, particularly if the tank-type heaters are kept below 60°C (140°F).

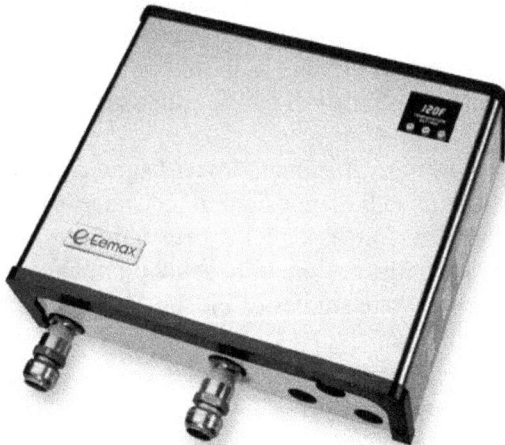

Tankless water heater. *Picture courtesy Eemax Inc.*

Maintaining your water heater

If you have a tank-type water heater, you (or a plumber) should drain and clean it annually to remove sediment and, to the extent possible, scale (hard water deposits). The annual cleanings will likely extend the life of the water heater in addition to minimizing conditions for *Legionella* growth. Follow the manufacturer's instructions to avoid damaging the heater or voiding the warranty.

Water softeners

If you have hard water, consider installing a water softener or electronic frequency water conditioner to minimize the build-up of scale in your piping.

Water softeners may lower *Legionella* risk also by reducing the amount of iron (which promotes *Legionella* growth) in the water. Most water softeners reduce iron by approximately 2 parts per million (ppm), which is probably sufficient for most public water supplies.

Don't rely on water softeners to lower *Legionella* risk by reducing calcium and magnesium in the water. Although one study indicated an association between *Legionella* and calcium and magnesium in hospital plumbing systems, two separate studies of Pittsburgh homes found no such association.

A possible but as yet unproven disadvantage of water softeners is their potential for serving as a habitat for *Legionella* growth.

What you need to know about water filters

Refrigerator and icemaker filters

Carbon or sediment filters typically used on lines supplying refrigerator icemakers and water dispensers, as well as most faucet and shower filters, provide a good habitat for *Legionella* and other bacteria. It's fine to use these filters to remove chlorine at the point of use, but be sure to replace them at the intervals recommended by the manufacturer, or sooner. Otherwise bacteria that build up on the filters may be released into the water.

Whole house water filters

Be careful about using whole house sediment or carbon filters. Both can provide a habitat for *Legionella*, and carbon filters also remove the disinfectant (chlorine, chloramines, chlorine dioxide) from the public water supply. If the filters are used, be sure to maintain them according to the manufacturer's recommendations.

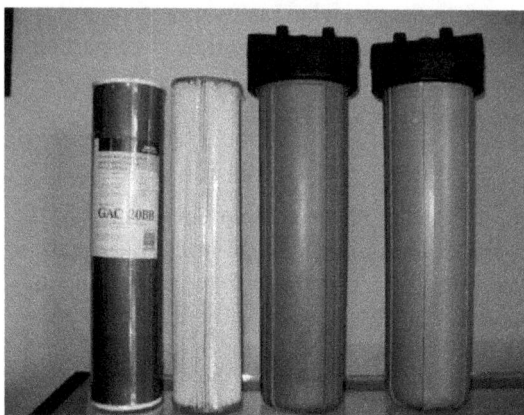

Filters (left) and filter housings

Humidifiers

Humidifiers are used to relieve dryness in the nose, throat, lips, and skin and to alleviate nuisances such as static electricity, peeling wallpaper, and cracks in paint and furniture.

Four types of humidifiers are marketed and sold today:

- Ultrasonic: Sound vibrations produce a cool mist.

- Impeller: A high-speed rotating disk produces a cool mist.

- Evaporative: A fan blows air through a wet wick, belt, or filter, transmitting moisture to the air.

- Steam vaporizer: Water is heated, releasing steam. "Warm mist" steam vaporizers cool the steam before it exits the machine.

Ultrasonic and impeller humidifiers generally pose a greater risk than do evaporative and steam units. Ultrasonic and impeller humidifiers efficiently disperse water particles into the air, whereas evaporative and steam humidifiers produce little airborne water particles. Also, *Legionella* and other bacteria are less likely to grow in steam humidifiers because of the high temperature.

Console humidifiers are encased in cabinets and placed on the floor. Portable humidifiers are smaller and easy to move. Central humidifiers are built into heating and air-conditioning ductwork for humidification of the whole house.

Portable humidifiers

Portable humidifiers have been blamed for cases of Legionnaires' disease and one study showed *Legionella* bacteria dispersed by a humidifier caused the disease in guinea pigs.

Do not use portable humidifiers or vaporizers unless absolutely necessary. If you must use them, take the following precautions:

- *Fill the humidifier with sterile water.* You can produce sterile water by boiling tap water for 10 minutes. Distilled water is second best. Do not use tap water. Tap water is more likely than distilled water to contain *Legionella.* In addition, minerals in tap water cause scale build-up in humidifiers, which can lead to microbial growth. Distilled water has fewer minerals than tap water, even tap water that has been treated by deionization or reverse osmosis. Be aware that water labeled "purified," "spring," "artesian," or "mineral" is not the same as distilled.

- *Disinfect the humidifier before each use.* Use a brush or other scrubber to remove any scale or film that has formed on the sides of the tank or on interior surfaces (be sure the power cord is unplugged). Follow the manufacturer's suggestions for cleaning products or disinfectants. In the absence of specific recommendations, clean all surfaces with either a bleach solution or a 3% solution of hydrogen peroxide. Rinse the tank thoroughly with sterile or distilled water (not tap water). Because *Legionella* and other bacteria can multiply rapidly in humidifiers within 24 hours, you should disinfect the humidifier daily (or more frequently if children, older adults, or immunocompromised adults live in the home) if it is used continuously for more than one day.

- *Clean the humidifier at the end of each humidifying season or whenever it will not be used again soon.* Before storage, make sure all the parts are dry. Dispose of used demineralization cartridges, cassettes, or filters. Store the humidifier in a dry location.

- *Take precautions when using demineralization cartridges, cassettes, or filters supplied with or recommended for your humidifier.* While demineralization accessories can help reduce your risk of bacterial growth, the effectiveness of these devices varies widely. Additional research is needed to determine how well and how long these devices work. In addition, these devices can be a breeding ground for *Legionella* and other bacteria if dirt or minerals build up in them. Watch for the appearance of white residue, which would indicate that minerals are not being removed.

The above procedures may need to be modified for console humidifiers. Check the manufacturer's recommendations for details.

Humidifiers installed in ventilation ductwork

Do not install humidifiers in ductwork unless absolutely necessary. If you must have whole-house humidification, take the following precautions:

- *Use a steam humidifier instead of the cold-water type. Legionella cannot survive at the high temperatures at which steam units operate.*

- *If cold-water humidifiers must be used, be sure that they don't use recirculated water but are supplied directly from the cold water plumbing.*

- *Inspect humidifiers for leaks. Keep them leak-free.*

- *Clean humidifiers periodically with bleach or another chlorine-based solution capable of killing bacteria without damaging the humidifier.* Check the manufacturer's recommendations regarding cleaning procedures and products. In the absence of specific recommendations, use either a bleach solution or a 3% solution of hydrogen peroxide.

New home design and construction

Hot water recirculation

Consider designing the plumbing system to circulate hot water continuously. Tiefenbrunner's study found that homes with hot water recirculation systems were less susceptible to *Legionella* growth than homes without them. The installer must extend the recirculation line to the point farthest from the water heater.

Piping

Consider copper piping instead of plastic or steel. In two studies, copper resisted *Legionella* growth best. Steel was second best. Plastics varied by type, but were generally more prone to *Legionella* growth than was steel. Rubber was worst. Copper also resisted scale and biofilm formation better than other materials.

During construction

The plumbing contractor should keep pipes and fittings clean and dry before installation. Piping will ideally be delivered and stored with end caps to keep dirt and water out until installation. Also, your plumbing contractor can put a chlorine tablet in every length of pipe before installation, which will help disinfect the piping after it is filled with water. These tablets are available from plumbing supply stores.

Water treatment and filtration

Consider a water treatment or filtration system, either for the whole house or on certain faucets and showers, but be careful which one(s) you choose. Some filters block *Legionella* but others actually promote bacteria growth. Whole house filters are discussed briefly above. A book to be released late in 2010 discusses on home-water treatment and filtration in detail (see www.hcinfo.com).

Before you occupy the home

Perform a hot water flush as soon as you move in, or a day or two before, even if the plumbing contractor puts chlorine tablets in the pipes. The hot water flush procedure is described above.

Water sampling

To test for *Legionella*, a water sample is collected into a bottle from a faucet, shower, or hot water tank and the bottle is sent to a laboratory for analysis. A faucet can be sampled also by wiping the inside of the fixture with a swab and having the slime on the swab tested. Laboratory fees for *Legionella* tests are expensive, about US$100-$150 per sample.

Routine sampling of home water is unnecessary, particularly for healthy nonsmoking adults who are at low risk of contracting Legionnaires' disease. However, if a member of your household contracts the disease, you may want to test the water to determine whether the home may have been the source of the *Legionella* that caused it. Also consider testing the home if it is occupied by someone who is immunocompromised.

To properly test a home plumbing system for *Legionella,* at a minimum collect a hot water sample from the faucet or shower that is used most (master bedroom), the kitchen faucet, and the drain of the water heater. If your budget allows it, collect samples from additional faucets or showers, and collect cold water samples also.

If someone in your home contracted Legionnaires' disease, ask your health department if it will provide a *Legionella* test at no charge. If it will not, and if you want to consider testing the home yourself, ask it for a list of laboratories in your country that are qualified to test for *Legionella*. Some countries, including the United Kingdom (http://www.hpa.org.uk/eqa/legionella) and the United States (http://www.cdc.gov/legionella/elite-intro.htm), have programs that test laboratories on their proficiency in *Legionella* analysis.

Analyzing water samples for *Legionella* is a highly specialized process so select a laboratory based on its qualifications, instead of just looking for the lowest price. For a given sample, a highly qualified laboratory may detect *Legionella* while a less qualified one will not. Don't waste your money on unreliable test results.

In addition to checking qualifications, ask laboratories if they will provide instructions for collecting and shipping samples and interpretation of the test results.

Protecting yourself while gardening

Although the vast majority of reported cases of Legionnaires' disease have been caused by exposure to *Legionella*-contaminated water, some cases have been contracted in the handling compost or potting soils.

Numerous infections from *Legionella*-contaminated compost have been documented in Australia and New Zealand, and a few in the United States, Japan, Scotland, and other countries, most from the species *longbeachae*.

Legionella was found in 33 (73%) of 45 potting soil samples collected in Australia in 1989 and 1990, 26 of which were identified as *Legionella longbeachae*.

Warnings were issued years ago about the risk of contracting Legionnaires' disease by inhaling dust that gets stirred up while turning over compost or while removing it from bags. This year, however, doctors concluded that a 67-year-old man, who was described as previously fit and healthy, contracted Legionnaires' through a cut on his hand while working with compost contaminated with *Legionella longbeachae.*

Public health agencies in Australia and New Zealand have recommended the following precautions when dealing with compost:

- Read the warning labels (required in Australia) on bags of compost and potting mix.

- Avoid stirring up dust.

- Avoid inhaling dust.

- Dampen the soil or compost before use.

- Wear a dust mask that fits tightly over the nose and mouth.

After the 2010 report of the case that doctors thought was caused by compost in a hand cut, the Royal Horticultural Society recommended that gardeners wear gloves when handling compost or compost bags. Warning labels on compost bags also recommend wearing gloves.

Whether at home or elsewhere, if you suspect that you are at high risk of contracting Legionnaires' disease because of water quality or your health, you can reduce your risk by using bottled or boiled (boil vigorously for three minutes and set aside to cool) water for drinking and brushing teeth and, in general, avoiding water splattering, sprays, and mists. In any circumstance, do not panic but take smart steps to reduce your risk and see a doctor if you experience Legionnaires' symptoms.

Bibliography

Adeleke A, Pruckler J, Benson R, Rowbotham T, Halablab M, Fields B. 1996. Legionella-Like Amebal Pathogens–Phylogenetic Status and Possible Role in Respiratory Disease. Emerging Infectious Diseases 2. July-Sept.

Alary M, Joly JR. 1991. Risk factors for contamination of domestic hot water systems for Legionella. Applied and Environmental Microbiology 57; 2360-2367.

Alary M, Joly JR. 1992. Factors Contributing to the Contamination of Hospital Water Distribution Systems by Legionellae. Journal of Infectious Diseases 165; 565-569.

Allegheny County Health Department, Pittsburgh. 1993. Approaches to Prevention and Control of Legionella Infection in Allegheny County Health Care Facilities. Pittsburgh: the Department.

Arnow P, Chou T, Weil D, et al. 1982. Nosocomial Legionnaires' disease caused by aerosolized tap water from respiratory devices. Journal of Infectious Diseases 146; 460-467.

Arnow PM, Weil D, Para MF. 1985. Prevalence and significance of Legionella pneumophila contamination of residential hot-tap water systems. Journal of Infectious Diseases 152; 145-151.

ASTM. 1996. Standard Guide for Inspecting Water Systems for Legionellae and Investigating Possible Outbreaks of Legionellosis (Legionnaires' disease or Pontiac Fever). West Conshohocken, Pa.: American Society for Testing and Materials.

Auckland Regional Public Health Service (ARPHS). Fact Sheet–Legionellosis. Available at www.arphs.govt.nz/notifiable/downloads/legionellosis.pdf.

Barbaree JM. 1991. Controlling Legionella in Cooling Towers. ASHRAE Journal, June; 38-42.

Barrett B. Mar. 1994. Trends in Occupational Health and Safety. Industrial Law Journal; 60-64.

Beierle J. 1993. Dental Operatory Water Lines. California Dental Association J 21; 13-15.

Benkel DH, McClure EM, Woolward D, Rullan JV, et al. 2000. Outbreak of Legionnaires' Disease Associated with a Display Whirlpool Spa. International Journal of Epidemiology, 200:29:1092-1098.

Besch EL, Dart DM, Goldman RF, Horton RJM, Logsdon RF, McNall Jr. PE, McQuiston FC, Turk A, Woods JE. 1989. Legionellosis Position Paper. Revised and edited by Feeley JC, under the direction of the ASHRAE Environmental Health Committee. Atlanta: American Society of Heating, Refrigerating and Air-Conditioning Engineers.

Beyrer K, Lai S, Dreesman J, Lee JV, Joseph C, Harrison T, et al. 2007. Legionnaires' Disease Outbreak Associated with a Cruise Liner, August 2003: Epidemiological and Microbiological Findings. Epidemiology and Infection 135: 802-810.

Blake G. 1963. The incidence and control of bacterial infection in dental spray reservoirs. British Dental Journal 19; 413-416.

Brady MT. 1989. Nosocomial Legionnaires' Disease in a Children's Hospital. Journal of Pediatrics 115; 46-50.

Breiman RF. 1992. Modes of Transmission in Epidemic and Nonepidemic Legionella Infections: Directions for Further Study. Presented at the 4th International Symposium on Legionella. In: Barbaree JM, Breiman RF, DuFour AP, eds. 1993. Legionella: Current Status and Emerging Perspectives. Washington, DC: American Society for Microbiology; 30-35.

Brennen C, Vickers JP, Yu VL, Puntereri A, Yee YC. 1987. Discovery of Occult Legionella Pneumonia in a Long-Stay Hospital: Results of Prospective Serologic Survey. British Medical Journal 295; 306-307.

Brundrett GW. 1992. Legionella and Building Services. Oxford, England: Butterworth-Heinemann.

Butler JC, Fields BS, Breiman RF. 1997. Prevention and Control of Legionellosis. Infectious Diseases in Clinical Practice 6; 458-464.

Cabot A, Miller R, Micik R, Ryge G. 1971. Studies on dental aerobiology: IV. Bacterial contamination of water delivered by dental units. Journal of Dental Research 50; 1567-1569.

Castellani Pastoris M, Vigano EF, Passi C. 1988. A Family Cluster of Legionella Pneumophila Infections. Scandinavian Journal of Infectious Diseases 20; 489-493.

CDC. 1997. Transmission of Nosocomial Legionnaires' Disease. Morbidity and Mortality Weekly Report 46; 416-421. US Department of Health and Human Services, Public Health Service, Centers for Disease Control and Prevention.

Ciesielski CA, Blaser MJ, Wang WL. 1984. Role of Stagnation and Obstruction of Water Flow in Isolation of Legionella Pneumophila from Hospital Plumbing. Applied and Environmental Microbiology 49; 984-987.

Communicable Diseases-Australia. Web site of the National Centre for Disease Control/Communicable Diseases Network, Australian Department of Health and Aged Care, http://www.health.gov.au.

de Jong B, Zucs P. 2010. Legionella, Springtime and Potting Soils. Eurosurveillance 15;8.

Den Boer JW, Yzerman PF, Schellekens J, et al. 2002. A Large Outbreak of Legionnaires' Disease at a Flower Show, the Netherlands, 1999. Emerging Infectious Diseases 8;1:37-43.

EPA. 1991. Guidance Manual for the Compliance with the Filtration and Disinfection Requirements for Public Water Systems Using Surface Water Sources, March 1991 Edition, Parts One and Two, Appendix B, "Institutional Control of Legionella," pp. 201-206. Washington, DC: US Environmental Protection Agency. EPA. 1991. Use and Care of Home Humidifiers, Washington, DC: US Environmental Protection Agency.

Farr BM, Gratz JC, Tartaglino JC, Getchell-White SI, Gröschell DHM. Sept. 17, 1988. Evaluation of Ultraviolet Light for Disinfection of Hospital Water Contaminated with Legionella. Lancet; 669-672.

Fass RJ. 1993. Aetiology and treatment of community-acquired pneumonia in adults: an historical perspective. J Antimicrob Chemother 32; 17-27.

Fiehn N, Henriksen K. 1988. Methods of disinfection of the water system of dental units by water chlorination. Journal of Dental Research 67; 1499-1504.

Final Recommendations to Minimize Transmission of Legionnaires' Disease from Whirlpool Spas on Cruise Ships. Atlanta: US Department of Health and Human

Services, Public Health Service, Centers for Disease Control and Prevention. Mar. 1997.

Fiore AE, Kool JL, Carpenter J, Butler JC. 1997. Eradicating Legionella from Hospital Water. Journal of the American Medical Association; Nov. 5, 1997;1404-1405.

Fitzgibbon EJ, Bartzokas CA, Martin MV, Gibson MF, Graham R. 1984. The source, frequency and extent of bacterial contamination of dental unit water systems. British Dental Journal 157; 98-101.

Fraser DW, McDade JE. 1979. Legionellosis. Scientific American 241:4; 82-99.

Freije MR. 1996. Legionellae Control in Health Care Facilities: A Guide for Minimizing Risk. Solana Beach, CA: HC Information Resources Inc.

Freije MR. 2000. Home Humidifiers: Reducing Your Exposure to Harmful Bacteria. Solana Beach, CA: HC Information Resources Inc.

Frequently Asked Questions about Legionnaires' Disease. Website of the Infectious Disease Section, VA Pittsburgh Healthcare System Center, Pittsburgh, USA, http://www.legionella.org.

Garbe PL, Davis BJ, Weisfield JS, et al. 1985. Nosocomial Legionnaires' Disease: Epidemiologic Demonstration of Cooling Towers as a Source. Journal of the American Medical Association 254; 521-524.

Garibaldi RA. 1985. Epidemiology of community acquired respiratory tract infections in adults: incidence, etiology, and impact. Am J Med 78; 32-37.

Gilpin RW, Dillon SB, Keyser P, Androkites A, Berube M, Carpendale N, Skorina J, Hurley J, Kaplan AM. 1985. Disinfection of circulating water systems by ultraviolet light and halogenation. Water Research 19:7; 839-848. First presented in part at the 13th International Congress of Microbiology, 1982, and at the 2nd International Symposium on Legionella, 1983.

Goetz A, Yu VL. April 1991. Screening for Nosocomial Legionellosis by Culture of the Water Supply and Targeting of High-Risk Patients for Specialized Laboratory Testing. American Journal of Infection Control; 63-66.

Gomez-Lus R, Gomez-Lus P, Garcia C, Gomez-Lopez L, Rubio MC. 1992. Investigation and Control of Nosocomial Legionnaires' Disease in Zaragoza, Spain. Presented at the 4th International Symposium of Legionella. In: Barbaree JM, Breiman RF, DuFour AP, eds. 1993. Legionella: Current Status and Emerging Perspectives. Washington, DC: American Society for Microbiology; 281-283.

Green M, Wald ER, Dashefsky B, Barbadora K, Wadowsky RM. 1996. Field Inversion Gel Electrophoretic Analysis of Legionella Pneumophila Strains Associated with Nosocomial Legionellosis in Children. Journal of Clinical Microbiology 34; 175-176.

Greene KA, Rhine WD, Starnes VA, Ariagno RL. 1990. Fatal Postoperative Legionella Pneumonia in a Newborn. Journal of Perinatology 10; 183-184.

Gross A, Devine MJ, Cutright DE. 1976. Microbial contamination of dental units and ultrasonic scalers. Journal of Periodontology 47; 670-673.

Guidelines for Design and Construction of Hospital and Health Care Facilities. Washington, DC: The American Institute of Architects. 1996.

Hahné S, Salmon R, Mukerjee A, Pankhania B. Apr. 20, 2000. Legionella from Welsh hotel guests indistinguishable from humidifier isolates. Eurosurveillance Weekly.

Haley CE, Cohen ML, Halter J, Meyer RD. 1979. Nosocomial Legionnaires' Disease: a Continuing Common-Source Epidemic at Wadsworth Medical Center. Medicine (Baltimore) 90; 583-586.

Hanrahan JP, Morse DL, Scharf VB, et al. 1987. A Community Hospital Outbreak of Legionellosis: Transmission by Potable Hot Water. American Journal of Epidemiology 125; 639-649.

Heath CH, Grove DI, Looke DFM. 1996. Delay in appropriate therapy of Legionella pneumonia associated with increased mortality. European Journal of Clinical Microbiology and Infectious Diseases 15; 286-290.

Helms CM, Massanari RM, Wenzel RP, et al. 1988. Legionnaires' Disease Associated with a Hospital Water

System: A Five-Year Progress Report on Continuous Hyperchlorination. Journal of the American Medical Association 259; 2423-2427.

Hlady GW, Mullen RC, Mintz CS, Shelton BG, Hopkins RS, Daikos GL. Oct. 15, 1993. Outbreak of Legionnaires' Disease Linked to a Decorative Fountain by Molecular Epidemiology. American Journal of Epidemiology; 555-561.

Hoge CW, Breiman RF. 1991. Advances in the Epidemiology and Control of Legionella Infections. Epidemiologic Reviews 13; 329-340.

Horie H, Kawakami H, Minoshima K, et al. 1992. Neonatal Legionnaires' Disease: Histopathological Findings in an Autopsied Neonate. Acta Pathologica Japonica 42; 427-431.

Horwitz MA, Marston BJ, Broome CV, Breiman RF. 1992. Prospects for Vaccine Development. Presented at the 4th International Symposium on Legionella. In: Barbaree JM, Breiman RF, DuFour AP, eds. 1993. Legionella: Current Status and Emerging Perspectives. Washington, DC: American Society for Microbiology; 296-297.

HSC (Health and Safety Commission). 2000. Legionnaires' disease: The control of Legionella bacteria in water systems. Approved Code of Practice and Guidance (L8). Sudbury, UK: HSE Books.

Jernigan DB, Hofmann J, Cetron MS, et al. 1996. Outbreak of Legionnaires' Disease Among Cruise Ship

Passengers Exposed to a Contaminated Whirlpool Spa. Lancet, 1996:347:494-499.

Joly JR, Dewaily E, Bernard L, Ramsey D, Brisson J. 1985. Legionella and domestic water heaters in Quebec City area. Canad Med Assoc J 132; 160.

Joseph CA, Watson JM, Harrison TG, Bartlett CLR. 1994. Nosocomial Legionnaires' disease in England and Wales, 1980-92. Epidemiology and Infection 112; 329-345.

Kelstrup J, Funder-Nielsen TD, Theilade J. 1977. Microbial aggregate contamination of water lines in dental equipment and its control. Acta Pathologica, Microbiologica, et Immunologica Scandinavica. Section B, Microbiology; 85:177-183.

Kerttula Y, Leinonen M, Koskela M, Makela PH. 1987. The aetiology of pneumonia: application of bacterial serology and basic laboratory methods. J Infect 14; 21-30.

Lee TC, Stout JE, Yu VL. 1988. Factors Predisposing to Legionella Pneumophila Colonization in Residential Water Systems. Archives of Environmental Health 43; 59-62.

Leoni E, De Luca G, Legnani PP, Sacchetti R, Stampi S, Zanetti F. 2005. Legionella waterline colonization: detection of Legionella species in domestic, hotel and hospital hot water systems. J Appl Microbiol. 98(2):373-379.

Lepine L, Jernigan D, Wyatt B, et al. 1995. Use of Urinary Antigen Testing to Detect an Outbreak of Nosocomial Legionnaires' Disease [abstract J58]. In: Proceedings and Abstracts of the Interscience Conference on Antimicrobial Agents and Chemotherapy. Washington, DC: American Society for Microbiology.

Leverstein-van Hall M, Verbon A, Huisman MV, Kuijper EJ, Dankert J. 1994. Reinfection with Legionella Pneumophila Documented by Pulsed-Field Gel Electrophoresis. Clinical Infectious Diseases 19; 1147-1149.

Liu Z, Stout JE, Tedesco L, Boldin M, Hwang CC, Yu VL. 1994. Ultraviolet Light Irradiation of Potable Water for Legionella Colonization in a Hospital Water Distribution System. ASHRAE Transactions 100, Pt. 1.

Lowry PW, Blankenship RJ, Gridley W, Troup NJ, Tompkins LS. 1991. A Cluster of Legionella Sternal-Wound Infections Due to Postoperative Topical Exposure to Contaminated Tap Water. New England Journal of Medicine 324; 109-113.

Lück PC, Dinger E, Helbig JH, et al. 1994. Analysis of Legionella Pneumophila Strains Associated with Nosocomial Pneumonia in a Neonatal Intensive Care Unit. European Journal of Clinical Microbiology and Infectious Diseases 13; 565-571.

Maher WE, Hackman B, Plouffe J. 1992. Rapid Thermal Disinfection of Legionella-Contaminated Water with a Drip Coffee Maker. Presented at the 4th International Symposium on Legionella. In: Barbaree JM, Breiman

RF, DuFour AP, eds. 1993. Legionella: Current Status and Emerging Perspectives. Washington, DC: American Society for Microbiology; 273-275.

Mahoney FJ, Hoge CW, Farley TA, Barbaree JM, Breiman RF, Benson RF, McFarland LM. 1992. Communitywide Outbreak of Legionnaires' Disease Associated with a Grocery Store Mist Machine. Journal of Infectious Diseases 165; 736-739.

Makin T, Hart CA. 1992. Efficacy of UV Radiation for Eradicating Legionella Pneumophila from a Shower. Presented at the 4th International Symposium on Legionella. In: Barbaree JM, Breiman RF, DuFour AP, eds. 1993. Legionella: Current Status and Emerging Perspectives. Washington, DC: American Society for Microbiology; 255-258.

Marrie TJ, MacDonald S, Clarke K, Haldane D. 1991. Nosocomial Legionnaires' Disease: Lessons from a Four-Year Prospective Study. American Journal of Infection Control 19; 79-85.

Marston BJ, Lipman HB, Breiman RF. Nov. 14, 1994. Surveillance for Legionnaires' Disease in the Eighties: Risk Factors for Morbidity and Mortality Related to Infection with Legionella. Archives of Internal Medicine; 2417-2422.

Marston BJ, Plouffe JF, Breiman RF, File Jr. TM, Benson RF, Moyenudden M, Thacker WL, Wong K, Skelton S, Hackman B, Salstrom S, Barbaree J, the Community-Based Pneumonia Study Group. 1992. Preliminary Findings of Community-Based Pneumonia

Incidence Study. Presented at the 4th International Symposium on Legionella. In: Barbaree JM, Breiman RF, DuFour AP, eds. 1993. Legionella: Current Status and Emerging Perspectives. Washington, DC: American Society for Microbiology; 36-37.

Martin MV. 1987. The significance of the bacterial contamination of dental unit water systems. British Dental Journal 163; 152-154.

Mcentegart MG, Clark A. 1973. Colonisation of dental units by water bacteria. British Dental Journal 134; 140-2.

Mermel LA, Josephson SL, Giorgio CH, Dempsey J, Parenteau S. Feb. 1995. Association of Legionnaires' Disease with Construction: Contamination of Potable Water? Infection Control & Hospital Epidemiology; 76-80.

Millar JD, Morris GK, Shelton BG. Jan. 1997. Legionnaires' Disease: Seeking Effective Prevention. ASHRAE Journal; 22-29.

Muder RR, Yu VL, McClure JK, et al. 1983. Nosocomial Legionnaires' Disease Uncovered in a Prospective Pneumonia Study: Implications for Underdiagnosis. Journal of the American Medical Association 249; 3184-3188.

Muder RR, Yu VL, Woo AH. Aug. 1986. Mode of Transmission of Legionella Pneumophila: A Critical Review. Archives of Internal Medicine; 1607-12.

Muraca PW, Stout J, Yu VL, Yee Y. 1988. Legionnaires' Disease in the Work Environment: Implications for Environmental Health, American Industrial Hygiene Association Journal 49; 584-590.

Muraca PW, Yu VL, Goetz A. 1990. Disinfection of Water Distribution Systems for Legionella: A Review of Application Procedures and Methodologies. Infection Control & Hospital Epidemiology 7:2; 79-88.

Oppenheim BA, Sefton AM, Gill ON, et al. 1987. Widespread Legionella pneumophila contamination of dental stations in a dental school without apparent human infection. Epidemiology and Infection 99; 159-166.

OSHA. 1996. Technical Manual; Section II, Chapter 7. US Department of Labor, Occupational Safety and Health Administration.

OSHA. 1998. Legionnaires' Disease Risk for Workers in the Plastic Injection Molding Industry. US Department of Labor, Occupational Safety and Health Administration.

OSHA. 1991. Re-Entry Protocols for the Social Security Administration, Western Program Service Center, Richmond, California. US Department of Labor, Occupational Safety and Health Administration, Health Response Team.

Pedro-Botet ML, Stout JE, Yu VL. 2002. Legionnaires' Disease Contracted from Patient Homes: The Coming of the Third Plague? Eur J Clin Microbiol Infect Dis 21:699–705.

Plouffe JF, File Jr. TM, Breiman RF, Hackman BA, Salstrom SJ, Marston BJ, Fields BS, the Community-Based Pneumonia Incidence Study Group. 1995. Reevaluation of the Definition of Legionnaires' Disease: Use of the Urinary Antigen Assay. Clinical Infectious Diseases 20; 1286-1291. First presented in part at the 32nd Interscience Conference on Antimicrobial Agents and Chemotherapy, 1992.

Point/Counterpoint: Surveillance Cultures for Legionella, a debate between Victor L. Yu, M.D. and Robert F. Breiman, M.D., about the pros and cons of sampling water for Legionella. Recorded at the 1996 Annual Scientific Meeting of the Society for Healthcare Epidemiology of America.

Pravinkumar S, Edwards G, Lindsay D, et al. 2010. A Cluster of Legionnaires' Disease Caused by Legionella longbeachae Linked to Potting Compost In Scotland, 2008-2009. Eurosurveillance 15;8.

Quaresima T, Castellani Pastoris M. 1992. Infezioni da Legionella sp. nel Bambino. Rivista di Italian Pediatrics 18; 125-136.

Reinthaler FF, Mascher F, Stenzner D. 1988. Serological Examinations for Antibodies against Legionella Species in Dental Personnel. Journal of Dental Research 67; 942-943.

Reynolds KA. 1998. Should You Be Concerned about Pathogen Transmission in Dental Lines? Water Conditioning & Purification; March; 188-120.

Robert M, Barbeau J, Prévost A, Charland R. Dental Unit Water Lines: A propitious environment for bacterial colonization. Unpublished paper posted at http://www.q-net.net.au/~legion/Legionnaires_Disease_and_your_Den tist.htm.

Rogers J, Dowsett AB, Lee JV, Keevil CW. 1990. Chemostat Studies of Biofilm Development on Plumbing Materials and the Incorporation of Legionella Pneumophila. Rossmore, HW, ed. Proceedings of the 8th International Biodeterioration and Biodegradation Symposium, 458-460. Barking, UK: Elsevier Science Publishers, 1991.

Rosa F. 1993. Legionnaires' Disease: Prevention and Control. Troy, Mich.: Business News Publishing Co.

Schofield GM, Wright AE. 1984. Survival of Legionella Pneumophila in a Model Hot Water Distribution System. Journal of General Microbiology 130; 1751-1756.

Shelton BG, Flanders WD, Morris GK. 1994. Legionnaires' Disease Outbreaks and Cooling Towers with Amplified Legionella Concentrations. Current Microbiology 28; 359-363.

Shojaei M, Staat RH. 1997. Disinfection of Dental Unit Water Lines Using Hydroperoxide: Preliminary Data. Journal of Dental Research, Abstract 3372.

Standards Australia. 2000. AS3666, Air-Handling and
Water Systems of Buildings, Microbial Control. Sydney.

States SJ, Conley LF, Ceraso M, et al. 1985. Effects of
metals on Legionella pneumophila growth in drinking
water plumbing systems. Applied and Environmental
Microbiology 50; 1149-1154.

Steele TW, Moore CV, Sangster N. 1990. Distribution of
Legionella longbeachae serogroup 1 and other
Legionella in potting soils in Australia. Appl Environ
Microbiol 56;2984-2988.

Steele TW. 1993. Interactions between Soil Amoebae
and Soil Legionellae. In: Barbaree JM, Breiman RF,
DuFour AP, eds. Legionella: Current Status and
Emerging Perspectives. Washington, DC: American
Society for Microbiology; 140-142.

Stout JE, Yu VL. 1997. Legionellosis. New England
Journal of Medicine, Sept. 4; 682-687.

Stout JE, Yu VL, Lee YC, Vaccarello S, Diven W, Lee
TC. 1992. Legionella pneumophila in residential water
supplies: environmental surveillance with clinical
assessment for Legionnaires' disease. Epidemiol. Infect.
109; 49-57.

Stout JE, Yu VL, Muraca PW. 1987. Legionnaires'
disease acquired within the homes of two patients. Link
to the home water supply. Journal of the American
Medical Association 257; 1215-1217.

Stout JE, Yu VL, Muraca PW, Joly J, Troup N,
Tompkins LS. 1992. Potable Water as a Cause of
Sporadic Cases of Community-Acquired Legionnaires'
Disease. New England Journal of Medicine 326; 151-
155.
Straus WL, Plouffe JF, File Jr. TM, et al. 1996. Risk
Factors for Domestic Acquisition of Legionnaires'
Disease. Archives of Internal Medicine 156; 1685-1692.

Struelens MJ, Rost F, Maes N, Maas A, Serruys E. 1992.
Control of Nosocomial Legionellosis Based on Water
System Disinfection by Heat and UV Light: a Four-Year
Evaluation. Presented at the 4th International
Symposium on Legionella. In: Barbaree JM, Breiman
RF, DuFour AP, eds. 1993. Legionella: Current Status
and Emerging Perspectives. Washington, DC: American
Society for Microbiology; 253-254.

Tablan OC, Anderson LJ, Arden NH, Breiman RF,
Butler JC, McNeil MMl, the Hospital Infection Control
Practices Advisory Committee. 1994. Guideline for
Prevention of Nosocomial Pneumonia. Atlanta: US
Department of Health and Human Services, Public
Health Service, Centers for Disease Control and
Prevention.

Thacker SB, Bennet JV, Tsai T, et al. 1978. An
Outbreak in 1965 of Severe Respiratory Illness Caused
by Legionnaires' Disease Bacterium. Journal of
Infectious Diseases 138; 512-519.

Tiefenbrunner F, Arnold A, Dierich P, Emde K. 1993.
Occurrence and Distribution of Legionella Pneumophila
in Water Systems of Central European Private Homes.

In: Barbaree JM, Breiman RF, DuFour AP, eds. Legionella: Current Status and Emerging Perspectives. Washington, DC: American Society for Microbiology; 235-238.

Tiefenbrunner F, Arnold A, Taraboi E, Cernek U, Emde K. 1990. Occurrence of Legionella in single family homes and hotels. Proc. German Assoc. Hyg. Microbiol. (In German.)

Tiefenbrunner F, Arnold A, Taraboi E, Cerneck U, Emde K. 1993. Comparison of Different Detection Methods for Isolation of Legionella Pneumophila from Water Supplies of Alpine Hotel Resorts. In: Barbaree JM, Breiman RF, DuFour AP, eds. Legionella: Current Status and Emerging Perspectives. Washington, DC: American Society for Microbiology; 198-200.

Tobin JO, Dunnil MS, French M, et al. 1980. Legionnaires' Disease in a Transplant Unit: Isolation of the Causative Agent from Shower Baths. Lancet 2; 118-121.

Vickers RM, Yu VL, Hanna S, Muraca P, Diven W, Carmen N, Taylor FB. 1987. Determinants of Legionella Pneumophila Contamination of Water Distribution Systems: 15-Hospital Prospective Study. Infection Control 8; 357-363.

Wallensten A, Oliver I, Ricketts K, Kafatos G, Stuart J, Joseph C. 2010. Windscreen wiper fluid without added screenwash in motor vehicles: a newly identified risk factor for Legionnaires' disease. Eur J Epidemiol June 2010.

WHO. 2005. Legionellosis fact sheet. Available at http://www.who.int/mediacentre/factsheets/fs285/en/index.html. Geneva: World Health Organization.

Womack SJ, Liang KC, Ilagan NB, Weyhing BT, Planas A. 1992. Legionella Pneumophila in a Preterm Infant: a Case Report. Journal of Perinatology 12; 303-305.

Woo A, Yu V, Goetz A. 1986. Potential In-Hospital Modes of Transmission of Legionella Pneumophila: Demonstration Experiments for Dissemination by Showers, Humidifiers, and Rinsing of Ventilation Bag Apparatus. American Journal of the Medical Sciences 80; 567-573.

Yu VL. 1997. Prevention and Control of Legionella: An Idea Whose Time Has Come. Infectious Diseases in Clinical Practice, Sept.-Oct.

Yu VL, Beam Jr. TR, Lumish RM, Vickers RM, Fleming J, McDermott C, Romano J. 1987. Routine Culturing for Legionella in the Hospital Environment May Be a Good Idea: A Three-Hospital Prospective Study. American Journal of the Medical Sciences; Aug., 97-99.

Yu VL, Liu Z, Stout JE, Goetz A. 1993. Legionella Disinfection of Water Distribution Systems: Principles, Problems, and Practice. Infection Control and Hospital Epidemiology 14:10; 567-570.

Yu VL, Plouffe JF, Castellani-Pastoris M, et al. 2002. Distribution of Legionella Species and Serogroups Isolated by Culture in Patients with Sporadic

Community-Acquired Legionellosis: An International Collaborative Survey. The Journal of Infectious Diseases 186:127–8.

Zuravleff J, Yu V, Shonnard J, Rihs J, Best M. 1983. Legionella Pneumophila Contamination of a Hospital Humidifier: Demonstration of aerosol transmission and subsequent subclinical infection in exposed guinea pigs. American Review of Review of Respiratory Disease 128: 657-661.

Please email your comments about this book, including suggested changes or additions, to hcinfo@hcinfo.com.

Thank you!

www.ingramcontent.com/pod-product-compliance
Lightning Source LLC
Chambersburg PA
CBHW071054280326
41928CB00050B/2508